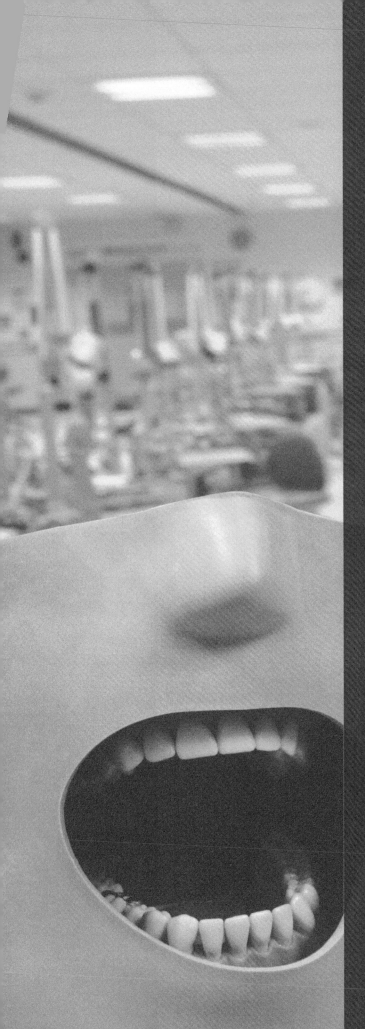

T0257021

Pre-Clinical
Dental Skills
at a Glance

I would like to dedicate this book to Claire for her love, support and encouragement; and to our two boys, George and Charlie.

I wish to thank my colleagues at Newcastle School of Dental Sciences for their input and support. I would also like to thank my students who, over a number of years, have provided invaluable feedback that guided the development of the book.

This title is also available as an e-book.
For more details, please see
www.wiley.com/buy/9781118766675
or scan this QR code:

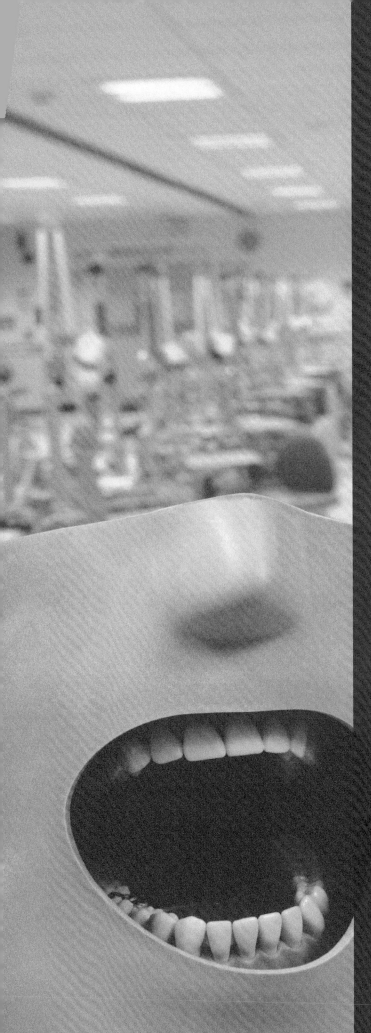

Pre-Clinical Dental Skills
at a Glance

James Field

BSc(Hons) BDS MFDS RCSEd MFGDP RCSEng
CertClinEd MA(Ed) SFHEA FAcadMEd PhD
Lecturer in Restorative Dentistry
School of Dental Sciences
Newcastle University
Newcastle upon Tyne, UK

WILEY Blackwell

This edition first published 2016 © 2016 by John Wiley & Sons Ltd.

Registered office:	John Wiley & Sons, Ltd, The Atrium, Southern Gate, Chichester, West Sussex, PO19 8SQ, UK
Editorial offices:	9600 Garsington Road, Oxford, OX4 2DQ, UK
	The Atrium, Southern Gate, Chichester, West Sussex, PO19 8SQ, UK
	1606 Golden Aspen Drive, Suites 103 and 104, Ames, Iowa 50010, USA

For details of our global editorial offices, for customer services and for information about how to apply for permission to reuse the copyright material in this book please see our website at www.wiley.com/wiley-blackwell

Library of Congress Cataloging-in-Publication Data
Field, James, 1979- , author.
 Pre-clinical dental skills at a glance/James Field.
  p. ; cm.
 Includes bibliographical references and index.
 ISBN 978-1-118-76667-5 (pbk.)
 I. Title.
 [DNLM: 1. Tooth Diseases–diagnosis.   2. Tooth Diseases–therapy. WU 140]
 RK305
 617.6'3–dc23
                                                                    2014047535

A catalogue record for this book is available from the British Library.

Wiley also publishes its books in a variety of electronic formats. Some content that appears in print may not be available in electronic books.

Set in Minion Pro 9.5/11.5 by Aptara

Printed and bound by CPI Group (UK) Ltd, Croydon, CR0 4YY

C9781118766675_080723

Contents

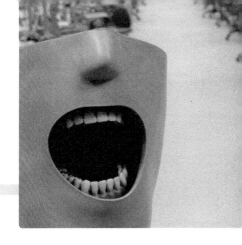

Preface

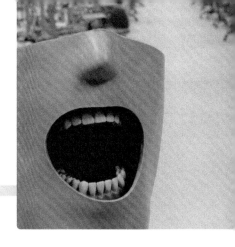

During most basic skills courses, you will necessarily make a significant and marked transition towards becoming an autonomous healthcare professional, working well within a clinical team and upholding professional and moral values. This is a tough journey, and sometimes it has to happen in little over three months. With the support and direction of your clinical teachers, this journey can nevertheless prove to be very rewarding.

This book is not a guide for established practitioners; it has been written primarily for pre-clinical students who are studying dentistry or dental-related subjects. It may also be useful as a revision aid for those preparing for basic skills-based assessments. A number of the handpiece exercises are conceptual rather than being based on modern clinical approaches; this will allow you to take a standardised and more consistent approach while you develop your basic skills. Furthermore, it will allow your clinical teachers to make more valid judgements about your decision making and operative control while in the skills lab.

Each chapter is limited to two pages in order to introduce the concepts concisely and to keep the guide simple and accessible.

Most of the figures are derived from teaching materials that I use within the skills lab, and they have undergone several iterations over the years. As such, I hope that they contain the detail necessary to support conceptual understanding without overburdening you with technical details. Clinical photos are kept to a minimum to avoid you *copying* a clinical endpoint; rather, you should be able to *visualise* a clinical endpoint based on your understanding of the approach. It is only then that you will be able to apply your skills more widely and deal with complications effectively. While this guide is intended to provide a very basic understanding of each skill, there are suitable suggestions for further reading for each chapter.

Surgical and soft tissue skills such as tooth extractions and administering local anaesthetic are not discussed in the book. Nonetheless, the chapters cover a comprehensive range of basic clinical operative and practical skills that should act as a sound framework on which to build.

James Field

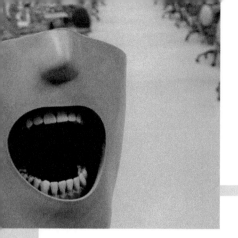

How to use your revision guide

Features contained within your revision guide

Each topic is presented in a double-page spread with clear, easy-to-follow diagrams supported by succinct explanatory text.

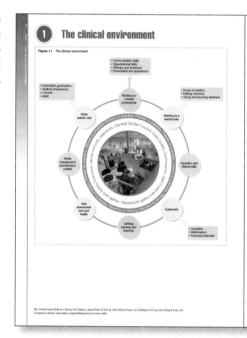

Your textbook is full of **photographs and illustrations**.

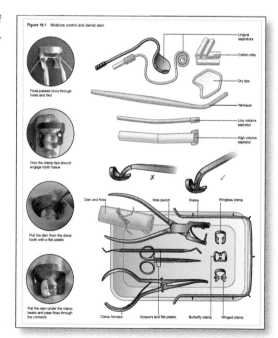

About the companion website

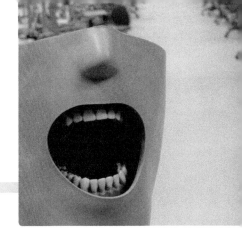

Don't forget to visit the companion website for this book:

www.wiley.com/go/field/preclinical-dental-skills

There you will find Extended Matching Questions for every chapter which have been specially designed to enhance your learning.

Scan this QR code to visit the companion website:

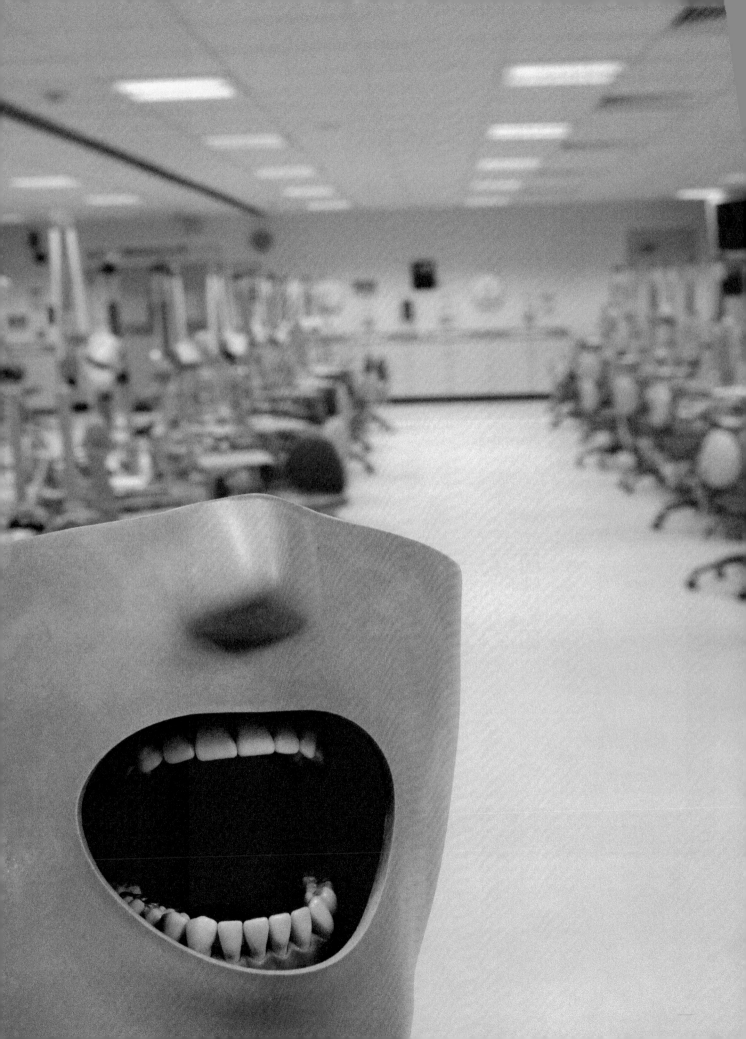

The clinical environment

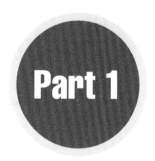

Part 1

Chapters

1 The clinical environment

Figure 1.1 The clinical environment

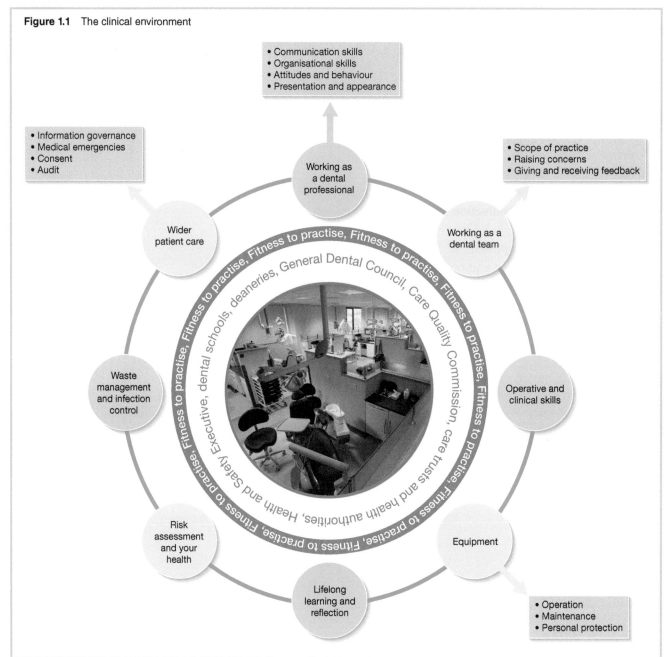

- Communication skills
- Organisational skills
- Attitudes and behaviour
- Presentation and appearance

- Information governance
- Medical emergencies
- Consent
- Audit

- Scope of practice
- Raising concerns
- Giving and receiving feedback

Working as a dental professional

Wider patient care

Working as a dental team

Waste management and infection control

Operative and clinical skills

Risk assessment and your health

Equipment

Lifelong learning and reflection

Fitness to practise, Fitness to practise, Fitness to practise, Fitness to practise, General Dental Council, Care Quality Commission, care trusts and health authorities, Health and Safety Executive, dental schools, deaneries, Fitness to practise, Fitness to practise, Fitness to practise, Fitness to practise

- Operation
- Maintenance
- Personal protection

Pre-Clinical Dental Skills at a Glance, First Edition. James Field. © 2016 by John Wiley & Sons, Ltd. Published 2016 by John Wiley & Sons, Ltd.
Companion website: www.wiley.com/go/field/preclinical-dental-skills

Entering the clinical environment as a healthcare professional should be a stimulating and rewarding experience. There is no doubt that it also requires a significant amount of preparation and training. It is a privilege that comes with a number of important obligations; you will carry out your own professional responsibilities as well as being responsible for engaging with, and often managing, the wider dental team.

Regulation

The way in which you work within the clinical environment will be governed by several regulatory bodies – their aim is to ensure optimal safety and patient care. It is your responsibility to make sure that you are adequately trained and competent in order to treat patients – this is known as 'fitness to practise'. The General Dental Council is the senior body that regulates dental professionals in the United Kingdom. However, other organisations such as academic institutions and statutory bodies will also take a career-long interest in your fitness to practise as you move through your training and into the workplace.

No doubt it is difficult enough to learn the basic skills necessary in order to treat patients operatively, but in isolation these skills are not enough to ensure the care and well-being of your patient base, or the efficiency and harmony of the dental team. When all is considered, the clinical environment has the potential to be complex and diverse. It is at this stage of your educational career when you must make sure that you are sufficiently organised and prepared to maximise the learning experience and drive your own learning. This may seem like a frustrating distraction for some people, but it will form a sound basis for lifelong learning and continued professional development.

Figure 1.1 outlines some of the important components and regulatory bodies with which you will need to engage in order to make an appropriate transition to clinical dentistry.

At the present time, the General Dental Council document 'Standards for the Dental Team' outlines nine principles that should underpin your practice, including:

- Putting patients' interests first
- Communicating effectively with patients
- Obtaining valid consent
- Maintaining and protecting patients' information
- Working with colleagues in a way that is in patients' best interests
- Maintaining, developing and working within your professional knowledge and skills
- Raising concerns if patients are at risk
- Making sure your personal behaviour maintains patients' confidence in you and the dental profession

You will also be expected to engage with clinical governance. This concept was introduced by the National Health Service in order to promote high standards of care, transparency, accountability and continual improvement in the delivery of care. The elements of clinical governance are often referred to as the 'seven pillars':

- Education and training
- Clinical audit
- Clinical effectiveness
- Research and development
- Openness
- Risk management
- Information management

Arguably, one of the most important elements of early professional development is adopting an appropriate attitude towards patient care and the dental team. Part of this is about how you appear to your patients and the wider public in terms of your behaviour, your appearance and how you communicate. As a student you are expected to make full use of your learning environment, which includes attending all the lectures, practicals and seminars that your institution provides for you. You are also expected to be punctual and to inform relevant individuals about planned or unplanned absences.

As a registered dental care professional, you will be expected to lead and manage at least part of the dental team. Aside from the above requirements, there will undoubtedly be a number of local guidelines, rules and regulations to adhere to; you should lead by example in this respect.

Personal protective equipment

For your own safety you will be required to wear personal protective equipment (PPE) in the form of eye protection, face mask and gloves. This also helps to convey an image of professionalism to the patient and the wider team within which you work. Safety glasses must be worn while using any cutting or rotary instruments, and while dispensing materials. Gloves should be used while in contact with the patient and their immediate environment, while handling clinical materials and when cleaning or disposing of dirty instruments. Face masks should be worn over the mouth *and* nose while using rotary instruments and working operatively on the patient. Your employer should provide reusable items of PPE, but within an academic institution you may be required to provide your own. Safety glasses should conform to safety standard EN166B/EN166A.

Uniforms and appearance

It is nearly always a requirement to conform to a dress code or uniform and appearance policy while working in a clinical environment. The main purpose of such a policy is to reinforce a professional image and to act as a barrier for personal protection and cross-infection control. Many policies stipulate a 'bare below the elbow' requirement; if you are in any doubt about what you can or cannot wear, then you must seek guidance from a senior clinical colleague, or obtain a copy of the policy yourself. It is also inappropriate to wear clinical attire outside of the clinical environment. You may be required to wash and maintain your own uniform.

In terms of your appearance, hair should be neat and tidy, secured from the face and lifted if longer than shoulder length. This is primarily to ensure your safety during clinical and laboratory procedures. Some policies will also stipulate requirements for the removal of jewellery. When considering hair colour and tattoos, please consider the patient base and dental team with which you are interacting in order to avoid causing any offence.

Dental loupes

Finally, many students ask me whether they should obtain their own set of dental loupes at this stage. I would recommend trying without these initially; basic dental procedures should not require any magnification and evidence suggests that there is no improvement in the operative performance of dental students. Loupes can, however, improve your posture, as they require you to work within a prescribed 'working distance'. If you decide to go ahead, it is critical that you obtain an appropriate prescription and that you have the opportunity to try the loupes before you buy them. There are many systems available, including through-the-lens, flip-up lens and illuminated loupes; each offers its own advantages. Higher magnification is not always better, and the field of view is an important consideration.

2 Lifelong learning and reflection

Figure 2.1 Lifelong learning and reflection

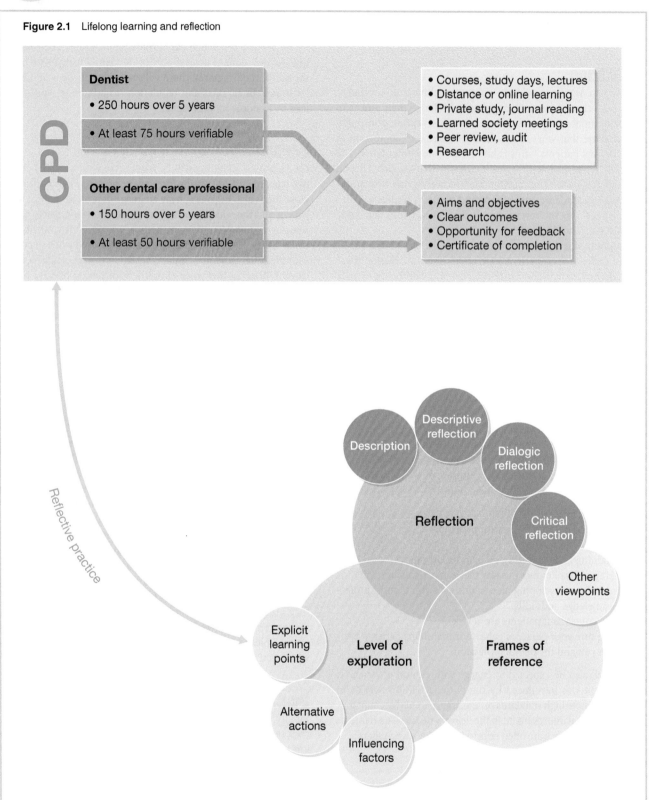

Lifelong learning

As a registered healthcare professional, you will have a duty to keep your skills and knowledge up to date throughout your career. This will ensure optimal patient care and confidence and, in addition, a regular and long-term commitment to learning. This approach is referred to as continuing professional development (CPD). The General Dental Council (GDC) requires you to plan, record and demonstrate evidence of this activity in order to remain on the practising register. Dentists should demonstrate 250 hours of activity over 5 years, with at least 75 of those hours being verifiable. You may also be asked to provide evidence of your CPD by other organisations, especially if you are undertaking a recognised training pathway, or as part of a professional development review or appraisal.

Support for learning

While you are in higher education it is easy to take for granted the resources available to you, such as paper books and e-books, journal access, study space and a defined curriculum. Mostly these are provided by your institution, although others may be available through memberships of associations or learned societies. Once you qualify, accessing learning resources becomes distinctly more difficult, both in terms of time and cost; as a result, many practitioners prefer to attend professional development courses where much of the legwork has been done already. At this stage it is important for you to be able to evaluate critically the resources available to you, and engage with activities that will benefit your own professional development.

Formats and subjects

General CPD may comprise courses and lectures, distance learning, private study, journal reading, multimedia learning, foundation training study days, learned society meetings, peer review, clinical audit and research. To be classed as verifiable activity, it must have concise educational aims and objectives, clear anticipated outcomes, quality controls (the opportunity for you to leave feedback) and documentary proof detailing the topic and number of hours of activity, along with your name and registration number.

CPD activity should cover subjects and topics that will benefit you professionally. This means that you are often left to use your own judgement. This is where a professional development plan becomes useful, so that you can show that you have not only satisfied the requirements, but also ensured that the activities are useful in your career progression. The GDC lists three core subjects and you are strongly encouraged to ensure that these are satisfied within the five-year cycle:

- Medical emergencies (10 hours)
- Disinfection and decontamination (5 hours)
- Radiography and radiation protection (5 hours)

Other recommended topics include legal and ethical issues, complaints handling and oral cancer: improving early detection.

Dental technicians are able to substitute radiography and radiation for materials and equipment-based topics.

Whatever CPD you undertake, it is important to get into the habit of making a record. This is known as a CPD log, and it will allow you to keep track of what you have carried out and what you still need to do.

Reflection

While lifelong learning ensures that you maintain the knowledge and skills you require for safe and effective patient care, the process of reflection informs and underpins that process. It allows you to analyse and evaluate your clinical experiences and, in its simplest sense, it presents a learning opportunity. In order to ensure that this process is effective, it is necessary for you to understand what reflection means. It is a skill that some people find easy to adopt, others less so. Regardless, it is a skill that you will refine over time. As an undergraduate, or for components of postgraduate assessment, you may be asked to reflect on particular clinical experiences (often referred to as 'significant events').

There are three important components to reflective practice:

1 Reflection You must be able to summarise the events as they unfolded (description). It is important to provide reasons for why things happened (descriptive reflection), but also to allow yourself to consider your emotions and explore alternative reasons (dialogic reflection). Ultimately, you should try to account for the social and political contexts within which you had your experience.

2 Frames of reference While ensuring that you can recall and rationalise your experiences, it is also very important to be able to consider how the experience unfolded for those around you – for example the patient, a relative or other members of the dental team.

3 Levels of exploration Consider the factors, both personal and external, that influenced what happened. What other choices did you have and what would the consequences have been of those choices? Finally, consider how you felt about the experience and whether you have learned anything – will you do things differently in the future?

Reflection and professional development

Undergraduate students and postgraduate trainees are increasingly being given the opportunity to record their CPD experiences as part of an electronic portfolio. Alongside your clinical activity, this provides a powerful tool for professional development planning. Your own reflections should be confidential, but it is a good idea to record them in such a way that they can help to inform your Professional Development Plan when the time comes. We tend to remember events that have happened recently, but it is valuable to be able to view reflections from weeks or months gone by.

Simulator jaws

Figure 3.1 Comparing plastic and natural teeth

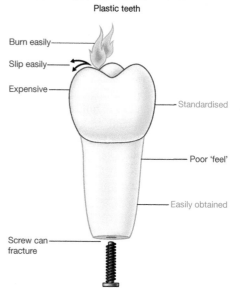

Natural teeth

Plastic teeth

Real feel

Hard to collect

Require cleaning and disinfection

Naturally retentive anatomy

Anatomically variable

Must remain hydrated

May be carious or fractured

Burn easily

Slip easily

Expensive

Standardised

Poor 'feel'

Easily obtained

Screw can fracture

Figure 3.2 Conceptual tooth anatomy

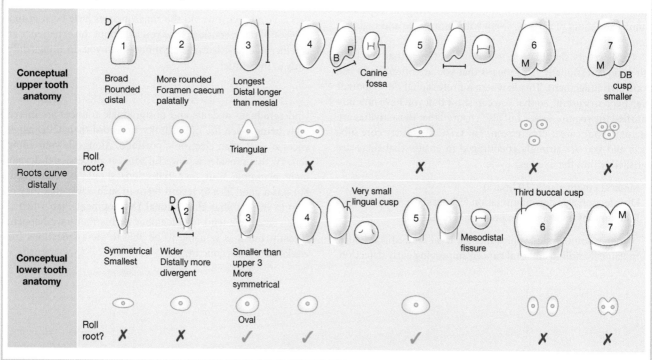

orking within a clinical simulation unit is vital in order to develop practical competence *and* a holistic approach to operative dentistry. The latter will necessarily include cross-infection control, posture, handpiece control, the use of lights and mirrors and the maintenance of equipment.

While you work as part of a wider 'team' in the skills unit, the simulator jaws themselves can provide a record of your own specific operative journey, involving skills such as preparations and intra-coronal restorations. Further courses may seek to develop skills for root canal treatment, extra-coronal preparations and implant placement or restoration. The clinical simulation unit and simulator jaws are also important tools for the assessment of these skills.

It is important for you to make the most of your time in this valuable environment; this is a rare opportunity to push the operative boundaries, take risks and (perhaps most importantly) critically reflect on these experiences.

Obtaining and storing natural teeth

Natural teeth are the preferred substrate for developing clinical skills. At present, simulator alternatives do not provide the same 'feel' of cutting enamel and dentine. Common problems include a lack of purchase on the enamel surface, resulting in the bur slipping; a tendency to burn more easily; and an inability to place adhesive restorations. It is also difficult to retain simulator teeth within the plaster jaw alongside their natural counterparts due to a lack of the complete root form.

It is becoming increasingly difficult to source unrestored and caries-free natural teeth, so collection from local practitioners and hospitals should be planned in good time. Consent is not required for material obtained from a living person that is to be used for educational or training purposes. It is important that the teeth are stored and transported appropriately – the teeth should be cleaned and stored in dilute hypochlorite (approximately 0.5%) in a hermetically sealed container. The solution should be changed at regular intervals (once every two weeks). It is a good idea to transport the containers in person to avoid the pitfalls of legislation relating to safe carriage. Obtaining teeth from abroad is not recommended, unless suitable ethical approval can be demonstrated from the country of origin.

The importance of tooth morphology

Setting up your own simulator jaw will allow you to begin to familiarise yourself with the relevant anatomical characteristics of each tooth type. Coronal morphology is important when both planning and placing a restoration. Unlike simulator teeth, natural teeth will display a variation in morphology. It is important to look very carefully at the presenting occlusal features such as the number and position of the cusps, the position and height of the marginal ridges, the fissure pattern, and whether there are large oblique ridges communicating the cusps and conferring particular structural durability. Knowledge of root morphology at this stage will help you to identify individual teeth and facilitate accurate tooth set-up. It is important to pay particular attention to the number and orientation of the roots, as well as their general curvature.

Terminology

From this point on, you must be familiar with the anatomical terminology of the teeth; it is used to communicate information within the patient records and to the wider dental team with consistency and clarity. Chapter 25 on charting the dentition provides more details.

Identifying teeth

Figure 3.2 is provided as a guide to help identify particular teeth. The following apply as a general rule.

- It is usually possible to roll the roots of the upper incisors, upper canines and lower premolars between the thumb and fore-finger.
- Upper molar teeth are usually three-rooted (two buccal and one large palatal) and lower molar teeth are usually two-rooted (mesial and distal).
- The lower first molar usually presents with five cusps (three buccal, two lingual) and the upper molars present with a noticeably larger mesial cusp.
- Tooth roots curve distally.

Important points for setting up and storing teeth

- The contact points of posterior teeth are not flat, nor are they positioned at the same height as the marginal ridge. Look carefully – they are lower than you think.
- Some teeth will be carious and therefore unusable within your simulator jaw, but take the time to look at where the caries exists and think about why.
- Look for large sweeping ridges across the occlusal surface, conferring structural durability – look to distinguish between large and accessory cusps that will help you to plan cavity preparations and restore.
- When natural teeth dry out they become brittle and crack more easily – ensure that you store the teeth wrapped in some damp gauze or paper towel.

Working within the simulator head

In the early stages of your technique course, it may be acceptable to work with only one arch of teeth installed within your simulator jaw. This gives you a little more space to develop your skills. Take care with the simulator cheeks, which will tear if stretched too far.

Advanced haptic systems

You may have the opportunity to work with haptic units for simulating handpiece use. These systems use virtual reality goggles and a stylus. Although fully simulated, they do allow you to work on a controlled and replicable scenario; this can be particularly useful if there is a need to standardise your work.

4 Basic restorative equipment

Figure 4.1 Types of restorative equipment

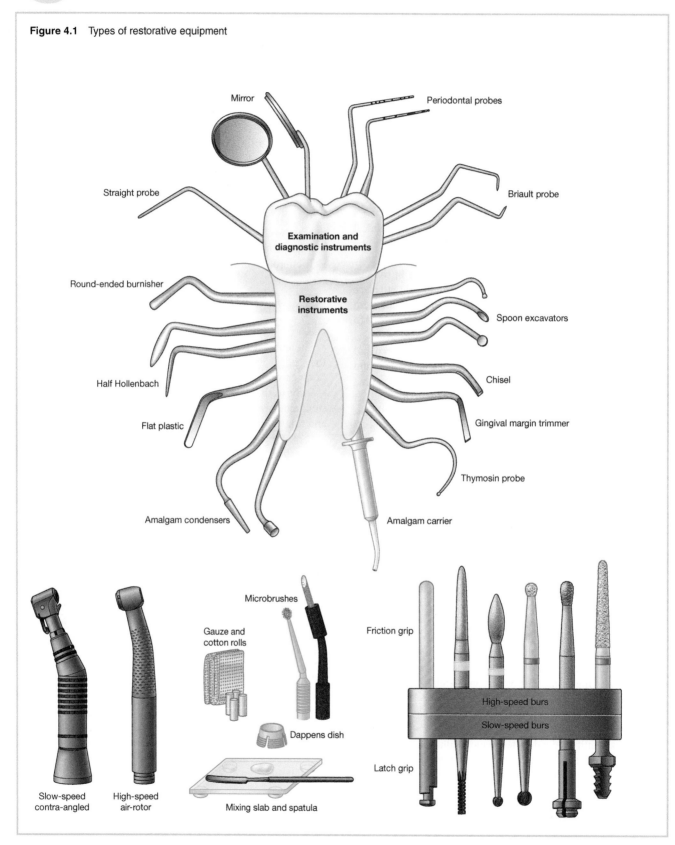

Pre-Clinical Dental Skills at a Glance, First Edition. James Field. © 2016 by John Wiley & Sons, Ltd. Published 2016 by John Wiley & Sons, Ltd.
Companion website: www.wiley.com/go/field/preclinical-dental-skills

Dentistry necessitates the use of a range of both hand and rotary instruments. Learning the instruments' names and their associated uses can be daunting at first. However, most of the basic equipment has stayed much the same for many years, and it is likely to remain so for the foreseeable future. It is important that you are able to choose the most appropriate equipment for each diagnostic, preventive and operative task. Often hand instruments are grouped into 'kits'. These may vary between institutions and even individual clinics; in primary care, kits are formulated mostly by clinician preference, but often in larger organisations, standard kits are constructed.

Examination instruments

Instruments used for examination and diagnosis are perhaps the most archetypal of all the hand instruments; namely, the dental mirror and the straight probe. Standard kits will also often include a periodontal probe and a Briault probe.

The *straight probe* is used for general exploration of surface texture and hardness. This is particularly important when assessing carious tooth tissue. This probe can also be used for crude exploration of depth and parallelism. It should (unsurprisingly) be straight and sharp. If not, it will at the least misrepresent surface features and lead to poor management of the carious lesion, often by cavitating early enamel lesions or underestimating carious activity within dentine. As with most hand instruments, a good finger rest is required to prevent unintentional (iatrogenic) damage to the soft tissues, especially the lips.

The *dental mirror* is used for indirect vision, but also (very importantly) for reflecting light to the operative field, and for retracting the soft tissues. Mirrors are available in two types: a front-faced single mirror and a double-surfaced mirror. In most cases the latter is used and is acceptable. You should ensure that the mirrored surface is free from significant scratches, otherwise this will distort your field of view. Mirror heads are often replaceable and so it is important to check that the mirror head is secured tightly to the handle. Disposable mirrors are also available, although these employ a plastic coating instead of glass and are easily distorted and scratched.

Periodontal probes are used for measuring attachment loss and assessing furcation involvement and bleeding on probing. The World Health Organisation (WHO) probe is colour-coded and ball-ended, and should be straight. The coloured bands refer to the Basic Periodontal Examination (BPE) gradings. The Williams probe is used for detailed data collection at specific intra-oral sites, and is marked in millimetre increments up to 10 mm.

The *Briault probe* is also used for general exploration of surface form, texture and hardness. As such, it should be sharp at both ends. It is a double-ended instrument and its shape means that it is particularly useful for exploring around tight corners or under margins. It is important not to exert a levering force with the Briault probe or it will easily distort; you should employ a good finger rest and be precise and definite with your movements.

Restorative hand instruments

Hand excavators (large, medium and oval) are particularly useful where judicious yet definite alteration of surface form is required, such as when carving mesial and distal pits into the occlusal surfaces of restorations or removing carious dentine directly over the pulp space. They should have sharp finished edges, and a good finger rest is essential to control the working depth of the instrument in a paring motion. The *straight or hatchet chisel* is used for removing unsupported enamel on the axial walls of a preparation. It should be employed parallel to the long axis of the tooth only, using a finger rest to avoid unnecessary fractures. *Gingival margin trimmers* have a curved blade with an oblique cutting edge for bevelling the base of interproximal preparations or rounding internal line angles. The *thymosin probe* is used for transporting thixotropic lining materials intra-coronally. The *amalgam gun* is used to dispense mixed amalgam into the tooth preparation; it is important to check that it works before you start and check that it is empty once you have finished dispensing; otherwise the amalgam will set within the chamber and the instrument will fail to work. *Condensers* are primarily used for packing plastic restorative materials, most often amalgam. Composite materials tend to stick to stainless steel instruments, so the *composite plastic* is gold-coated to facilitate manipulation of the material. The *Mortenson's condenser* is particularly useful for packing into deeper, less accessible areas of the preparation; its length also makes it a useful instrument for burnishing aluminium matrices. The *half Hollenbach* is primarily used for carving restorative materials. It is a double-ended instrument and the distinctive leaf-shaped cutting edges should (where possible) rest partially on natural tooth tissue to ensure that cusp and fissure form are restored accurately. *Round-ended burnishers* are useful for maintaining a smooth finish while manipulating materials; however, they can create marginal deficiencies and an overly shallow occlusal contour. *College tweezers* are very useful for transferring items to and from the mouth, most often cotton wool and gauze. The *flat plastic* is possibly the most ubiquitous instrument due to its flat and contra-angled heads. It should not be used as a lever or a screwdriver, nor is it ideal for carving restorative materials. Often a pair of *scissors* is particularly useful for trimming floss, matrices, cotton rolls, gauze and rubber dam.

Handpieces and burs

Basic skills courses are likely to introduce you to the high-speed air turbine (air rotor) and the slow-speed contra-angled handpiece. The air rotor is normally water-cooled due to its high speed of rotation, and uses a variety of diamond-coated or tungsten-carbide burs to cut through tooth tissue and other restorative materials. The slow-speed handpiece rotates much more slowly and, as such, requires more aggressive cutting surfaces from its stainless steel burs and mandrel attachments. Typically the slow speed would be used for cutting dentine and polishing restorative materials. The slower rotations create a more vigorous vibration (annoyance factor) than the air rotor.

Other equipment

A range of other standard items is shown in Figure 4.1, including mixing slabs, spatulas and dappen dishes. A selection of matrix bands are also available (celluloid or metal) with their respective matrix retainers. These are discussed further in Chapter 7.

5 Handpiece maintenance and operation

Figure 5.1 Handpieces

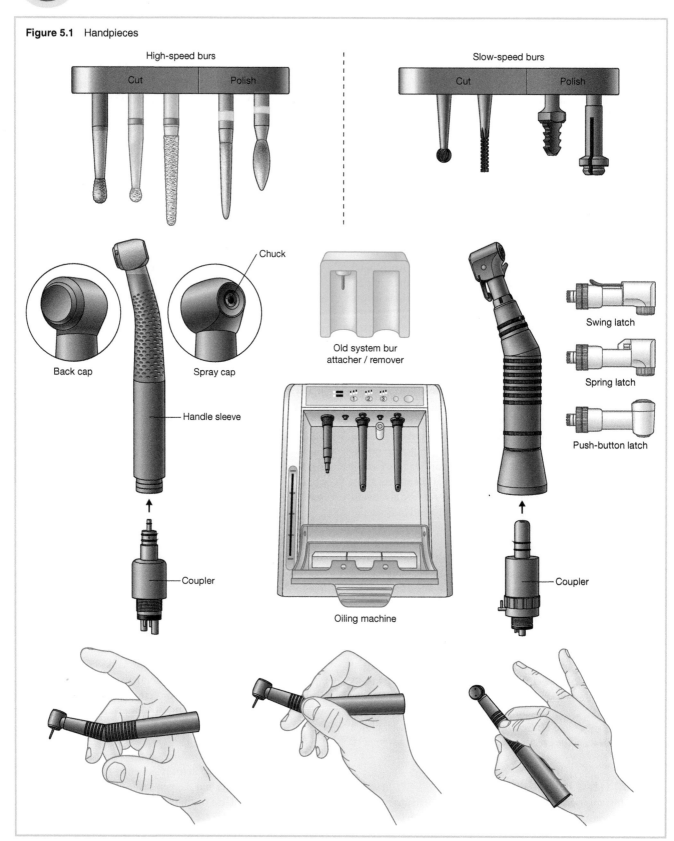

High-speed burs

Cut | Polish

Slow-speed burs

Cut | Polish

Chuck

Back cap

Spray cap

Old system bur attacher / remover

Swing latch

Spring latch

Push-button latch

Handle sleeve

Coupler

Oiling machine

Coupler

Pre-Clinical Dental Skills at a Glance, First Edition. James Field. © 2016 by John Wiley & Sons, Ltd. Published 2016 by John Wiley & Sons, Ltd.
Companion website: www.wiley.com/go/field/preclinical-dental-skills

Being able to use dental handpieces is undoubtedly one of the most exciting and anticipated moments for a pre-clinical dental student. Removal of tooth tissue is much more effective using rotary instruments than hand instruments, but make no mistake about the ease with which hard and soft tissues can be irreversibly damaged. The safe environment of a clinical skills laboratory provides the perfect opportunity for you to develop these skills before treating patients.

The two most commonly used handpieces are the high-speed air rotor (250,000–400,000 rpm) and the contra-angled slow-speed handpiece (500–25,000 rpm). Examples of other handpieces include:

- Straight handpieces
- Speed-reducing handpieces
- Torque-limiting handpieces
- Oscillating, ultrasonic and piezoelectric handpieces
- Air abrasion handpieces

The air rotor and slow-speed handpieces behave very differently to one another, primarily due to their speed of rotation. The air rotor's speed results in a smooth and accurate cutting performance while producing a loud and high-pitched noise. The speed also necessitates the use of water coolant to prevent overheating of the tooth surface.

The slow-speed handpiece is much quieter but displays greater eccentricity due to the lower speed; this results in a coarser cutting experience, with a greater degree of vibration.

Safe operation

Both types of handpiece need to be kept under fine control to prevent any unnecessary tissue damage. The high-speed handpiece has the potential to cut indiscriminately into hard and soft tissues, whereas the slow-speed handpiece has the potential to slip across the hard tissues, causing trauma to adjacent structures. These hazards can be reduced by:

- Holding the handpieces correctly
- Ensuring that an effective finger rest is used

Handpieces should be sterilised before use. Both the high- and slow-speed units should attach to the couplings with a positive click. Depending on the manufacturer, handpieces may simply pull away from the coupling to detach, or employ a release button or the retraction of a collar. It is important to ensure that the handpieces are positively connected; within the high-speed coupling there are connections for compressed air, water and often LED or fibre-optic lighting components. The rotating side of the high-speed handpiece should never be pointed directly at the face without adequate personal protective equipment, comprising safety goggles and a face mask.

It is possible to regulate handpiece speeds using either the unit control panel or the foot pedal. When cutting tooth tissue, the high-speed handpiece should be run at maximum power to ensure that water flow is sufficient and torque is maximal; only when polishing with appropriate burs should it be slowed down. When cutting intra-coronal preparations, you should never allow a handpiece to stop completely while working within the body of the tissue.

Hand holds and finger rests

The 'pen' grip is most appropriate for both the high-speed and contra-angled slow-speed handpiece (see Figure 5.1). It is important to identify the fingers to be used for resting (usually the fourth and fifth fingers). The thumb and forefinger should nestle in the divergence of the handle in order to act as a fulcrum about which the handpiece can move. Holding the handpiece closer to or further away from the head reduces the level of control. The finger rests can employ adjacent, contralateral or opposing hard tissues; however, the fingers should never rest on mobile tissues.

Checking the air rotor handpiece

The following components should be checked on every occasion the handpiece is unpackaged.

- Back cap secure
- Spray cap secure
- Friction grip chuck secure
- LED coverings intact
- Bearings not worn, causing burs to move erratically
- Handle sleeve secure
- Coupled correctly to the unit

Faulty handpieces should be set aside and dealt with promptly through a service provider or instrument curator.

Maintenance

Regular maintenance is important in order to ensure trouble-free and cost-effective operation. After use, handpieces should be cleaned and disinfected, avoiding glutaraldehyde or chlorine-based solutions. The handpieces should then be lubricated with service oil using a can or machine dispenser (see Figure 5.1) and packaged prior to sterilisation.

Burs and uses

All burs should conform to international standard ISO 6360 in terms of materials, dimensions and colour codings. It is critical that you are aware of the dimensions of the and its intended purpose. Many burs are now also single use and so it is important to check.

Most high-speed burs either chip (tungsten carbide) or abrade (diamond-coated) the enamel and dentine. Slow-speed burs often rely on stainless steel flutes with a positive rake to carve at the dentine; these will not remove sound enamel effectively. Mandrels are also available for slow-speed handpieces to mount polishing discs and brushes; be careful not to overheat the tooth surface, ensuring that you use short bursts of activity.

The burs should be secure within the handpiece, either with a friction grip (high speed) or a latch grip (slow speed). Finally, it is critical to ensure that that the slow-speed handpiece is operating in a forward direction, otherwise the bur flutes will fail to engage the tooth tissue correctly.

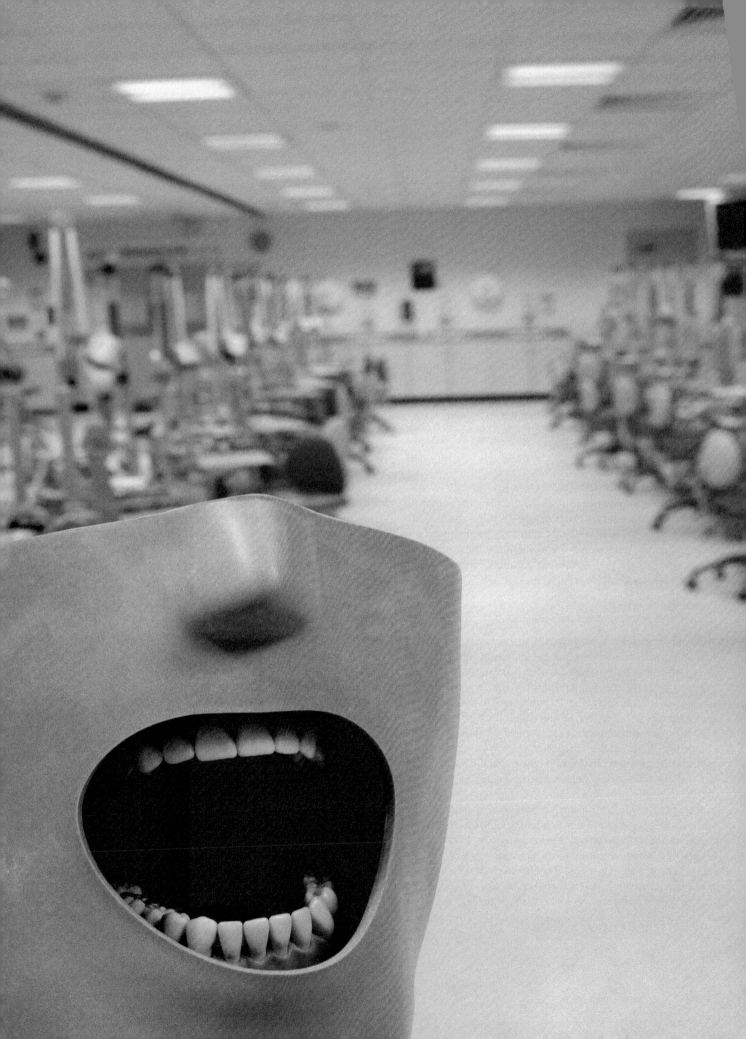

Basic operative skills

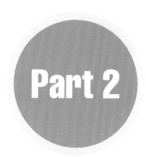

Part 2

Chapters

6 Posture and working with a dental mirror

Figure 6.1 Guidelines for posture

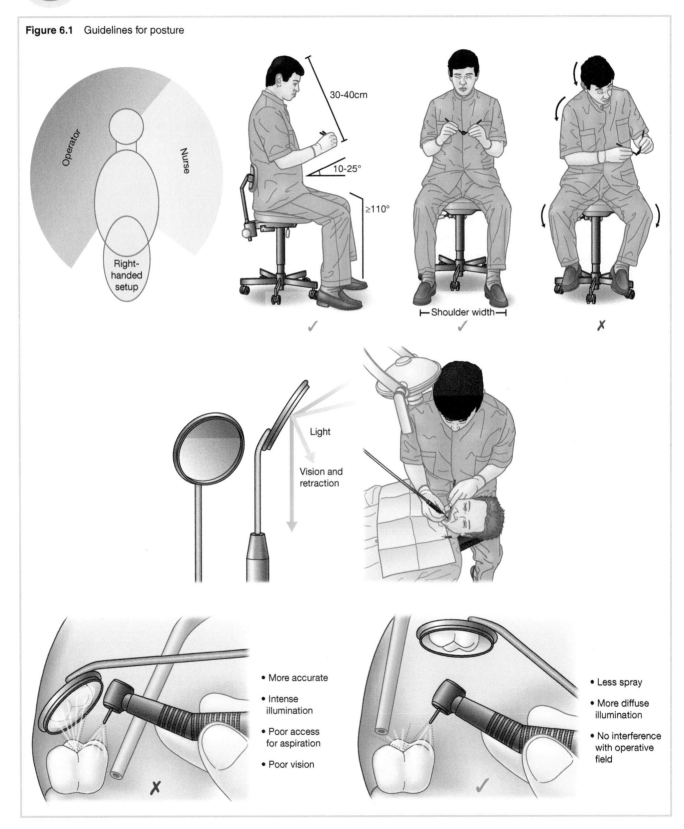

When you are operating on teeth for the first time, posture and patient positioning are often the last things on your mind. Nonetheless, it is really important to establish good habits from the very beginning, for two main reasons:

• Improved posture will ensure that you maintain a healthy back throughout your career.
• Paying attention to your posture and the patient's positioning will improve your access and direct visibility.

Achieving a good posture is one of the core dental skills that can benefit from peer review on an almost continuous and perpetual basis; it can be difficult when you are concentrating to be aware of your own posture, so don't be afraid to offer advice to or receive advice from colleagues.

The diagrams in Figure 6.1 propose designated working areas for you and your nurse, and ideal postures in relation to limb and head position. It is very important to make yourself comfortable in the operator chair first, before adjusting your patient.

Mirror work

Working in a mirror is a complex skill that takes much practice. Nonetheless, within the boundaries of a healthy operating position and patient positioning, you should be trying to work with direct vision whenever possible. When direct vision is not possible, try holding the dental mirror closer and further from your operative site. You will notice that the effects of debris and water spray are much reduced the further away the mirror is retracted; access for other instruments such as the high-volume aspirator is also improved. This mirror position is often at the expense of better illumination and magnification.

Make the most of the opportunity in the skills laboratory to try out different seating positions and patient postures. There are no hard-and-fast rules here – the aim is to find your own comfortable, healthy and effective way of working.

General seating position

It is important to ensure that you are sitting in a fairly relaxed position. You should be utilising the full area of the seat, which means pushing your bottom into the far corner rather than perching on the edge. Your back should also be straight – in a straight-backed chair this would mean that your middle back moves away from the support while your shoulders and lower back remain in line with your bottom. Over time, your body will fatigue and you will slouch. In an operative chair, the back rest should be adjusted to support the middle back, in order to help maintain the correct posture over a longer period. Some operative seats (such as saddle seats) have no back support; the theory here is that their forward tilt encourages you to keep a straight back. Key to this principle is that the seat should also enforce a semi-standing position, with the upper legs meeting the lower legs at ≥120 degrees.

Your upper arms should be held relatively close to your body, rather than being held out (think of a chicken flapping its feathers). The lower arms should be level with or angled slightly away from the floor. Your feet should be flat on the floor, about shoulder width apart, and the lower leg should be near enough vertical.

It is okay to bend forwards away from the back rest on the odd occasion, but try to keep this to a minimum. Similarly, most of the time the head should be maintained in a forward direction. Bending to the side and rotating the body and head are considered to be risky movements for your back and neck.

Fields of vision

Once you have positioned yourself comfortably, your attention should turn to the patient's position. Where possible you should be using direct vision, so it is important to remember that there are a number of options.

Directly behind the patient (12 o'clock position) – this is good for:

• Direct vision of the labial surfaces of the upper and lower teeth, the occlusal surfaces of the lower teeth and (with the patient's head tilted to the side) the buccal surfaces of the posterior teeth.
• Indirect vision of the palatal and occlusal surfaces of the upper teeth and the lingual surfaces of the lower teeth.

Moving around to the side (9 o'clock position) – this is good for:

• Direct vision of the ipsilateral buccal surfaces and the contralateral palatal and lingual surfaces (and vice versa for indirect vision).
• With the patient's head tilted slightly back and towards you, direct vision of the occlusal and interproximal operative surfaces of the posterior teeth.

Moving in front of the patient to face them (7 o'clock position) – this is good for:

• Direct vision of the labial surfaces and lower occlusal surfaces.
• Indirect vision of the lower lingual surfaces anteriorly.

The next aim is to position the light so that it is convergent with your field of vision. If direct, the light should be illuminating the actual operative surface; if indirect, the light should be illuminating the mirror face. On occasion it may be necessary to use the mirror to illuminate a directly visualised operative field, particularly if your instrument or choice of finger rest is casting an unfavourable shadow.

Dynamics and working with your nurse

Try to remember that you will be working with a dental nurse in due course, and they will also need to be positioned at the patient's side. Mostly this is to your non-dominant side – if you are right-handed this will be between the 12:30 and 3:30 clock positions. There are occasions when it is appropriate to swap over if access or visibility is proving to be difficult.

To reiterate, within the boundaries of a healthy operating position and patient positioning, you should be trying to work with direct vision whenever possible. This means adopting a dynamic approach, changing the patient's and your own positions as often as necessary.

7 Effective use of posterior matrices

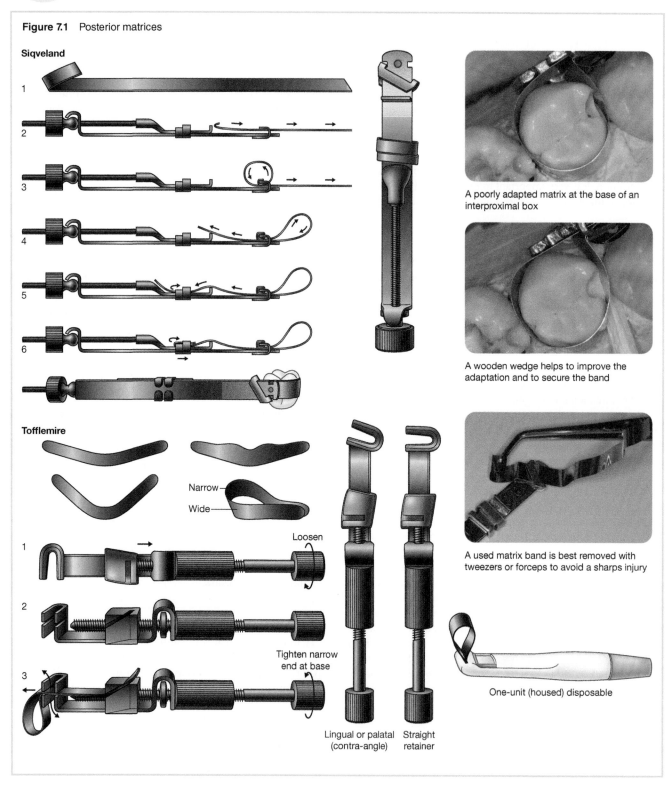

Figure 7.1 Posterior matrices

Siqveland

Tofflemire

Narrow

Wide

Loosen

Tighten narrow
end at base

Lingual or palatal   Straight
(contra-angle)   retainer

A poorly adapted matrix at the base of an
interproximal box

A wooden wedge helps to improve the
adaptation and to secure the band

A used matrix band is best removed with
tweezers or forceps to avoid a sharps injury

One-unit (housed) disposable

Pre-Clinical Dental Skills at a Glance, First Edition. James Field. © 2016 by John Wiley & Sons, Ltd. Published 2016 by John Wiley & Sons, Ltd.
Companion website: www.wiley.com/go/field/preclinical-dental-skills

When a direct restoration is intended to replace the proximal, lateral or medial aspect of a posterior surface, then there is a need to constrain the restorative material to within the circumference of the tooth. Matrices are extremely useful for this purpose, allowing the accurate placement of relatively small approximal preparations through to full cuspal replacements. Matrices should not be used in order to protect the adjacent tooth from iatrogenic damage while refining a preparation.

A variety of posterior matrices and retainers are available; all matrices are single use:

- Metal matrices in autoclavable metal retainers
- Metal matrices in single-use plastic retainers
- Metal matrices held in situ by interproximal clamps
- Cellulose matrices

Cellulose matrices are not recommended for posterior amalgam restorations, as it is not possible to exert adequate apical force in order to condense the material appropriately.

Interproximal wedges

It is imperative that a matrix is held in place interproximally using a wedge. This ensures good adaptation at the base of the preparation, and prevents excess restorative material from being displaced apically and causing a positive ledge. Once your matrix is in place, the level of adaptation should be checked carefully intra-coronally with a straight probe.

Wooden wedges are considered to be most suitable: rigid enough to support the matrix against the tooth surface, yet soft enough to be pushed adequately into the embrasure space and adapt to the tooth contour. Wooden wedges also act to separate the posterior teeth slightly, facilitating a definite contact point to the restoration. Care must be taken to ensure that the wedge is not overloaded otherwise it will snap, potentially leaving small fragments interproximally. Plastic wedges are available, but often fail to hold the matrix firmly against the tooth surface or separate the teeth to any useful degree, and they exhibit poor retention.

Matrix tips

Once a matrix is assembled, it is normally relatively easy to place it over the tooth. In some situations the contact can be particularly tight, so flossing interproximally first can help. Failing that, a wooden wedge can help to separate the teeth, but this will need to be withdrawn and replaced once the matrix is seated. The wedge will then separate the teeth slightly *and* help to hold the matrix in place. It is important at this stage to ensure that the matrix is contacting the adjacent tooth, otherwise you will fail to obtain a contact point. Metal matrices can be burnished up to the contact using the long axis of a straight instrument such as a Mortonson's condenser or even a straight probe. Cellulose matrices can be troublesome in this situation, and it may be necessary to reposition the matrix in order to develop a more passive contact point.

The matrix itself should sit at least 1.5 mm above the anticipated restoration in order that you can pack sufficient material into the preparation without compromising the integrity or form of the superficial margins. If the matrix is too narrow (even when using the widest matrix), then it may be necessary to consider placing a primary base to the restoration in composite or glass ionomer first, before raising the matrix and completing the full restoration. Alternatively, it may be appropriate to consider an indirect restoration if management is proving difficult.

The final basic consideration is the retainer position. Depending on the system being used, it may not be possible to place the retainer lingually or palatally without dislodging or deforming the matrix. This is particularly critical when restoring a large portion of the tooth on the buccal aspect; flexural forces on the matrix tend to pull the buccal aspect medially, flattening the final contour of the restoration. The Tofflemire system has a contra-angled retainer that facilitates placement lingually or palatally. With both the Tofflemire and Siqveland systems, the matrix is retained as a loop. As such, the confluence of the matrix may sit adjacent to an area of intended restoration. Where possible, it is best to avoid this situation, particularly when placing a composite restoration. With amalgam, the excess contour can be easily carved back after matrix removal.

Siqveland

The Siqveland system is very common and can be constructed with narrow and wide matrices. Assembly is relatively time-consuming and complex in comparison to other systems (see Figure 7.1), but the final assembly is undoubtedly more durable and stable. There may be difficulty with lingual or palatal placement of the retainer.

Tofflemire

The Tofflemire system can be constructed with universal, broad or narrow matrices. The latter two types are wider around the interproximal areas to account for deeper approximal box preparations. This system is quicker to assemble than the Siqveland, and the matrix can exit three ways from the retainer head, which can help to manage the band confluence more effectively. The contra-angled retainer can also be used lingually or palatally. Care should be taken to ensure that the matrix does not rotate out of the retainer.

Other systems

Matrices with interproximal clamps are available; although they are simple and quick to apply, the level of adaptation is compromised compared to retainer systems. It can be particularly difficult to condense effectively or ensure that the matrix is tight at the base; an interproximal wedge is essential with these systems. Housed (closed-unit) disposable retainers are becoming popular and will certainly reduce the risk of injury during placement and disposal.

Dismantling

Great care should be taken when disassembling matrices from reusable retainers. Forceps should be used and matrices dropped straight into a sharps bin.

Controlling bur depth and angulation

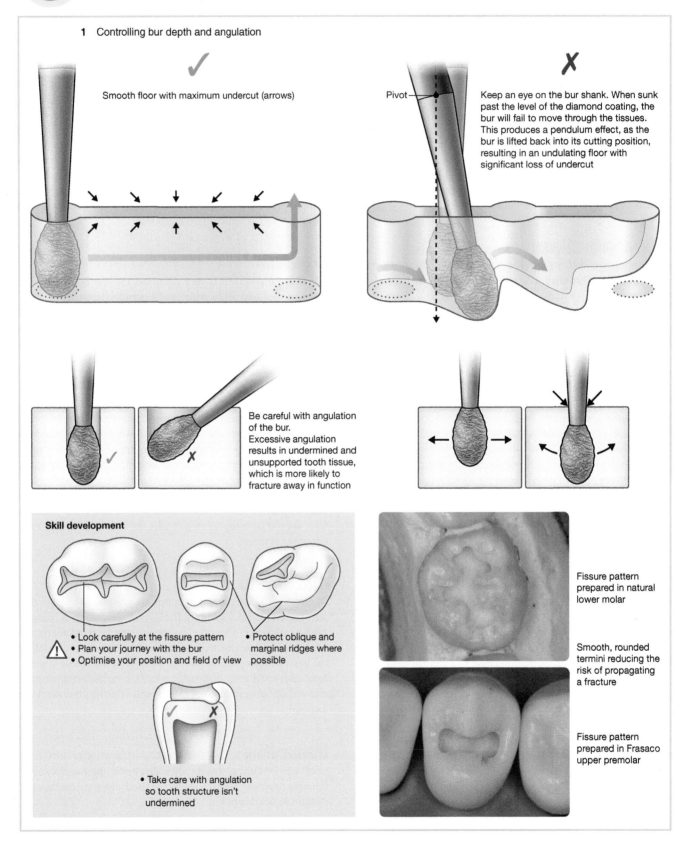

1 Controlling bur depth and angulation

✓

Smooth floor with maximum undercut (arrows)

✗

Pivot → Keep an eye on the bur shank. When sunk past the level of the diamond coating, the bur will fail to move through the tissues. This produces a pendulum effect, as the bur is lifted back into its cutting position, resulting in an undulating floor with significant loss of undercut

✓ ✗ Be careful with angulation of the bur. Excessive angulation results in undermined and unsupported tooth tissue, which is more likely to fracture away in function

Skill development

⚠ • Look carefully at the fissure pattern
• Plan your journey with the bur
• Optimise your position and field of view

• Protect oblique and marginal ridges where possible

✓ ✗

• Take care with angulation so tooth structure isn't undermined

Fissure pattern prepared in natural lower molar

Smooth, rounded termini reducing the risk of propagating a fracture

Fissure pattern prepared in Frasaco upper premolar

Once the decision for operative intervention has been made, it is important that tooth tissue is removed in a controlled and coordinated manner. When control is lacking, iatrogenic damage can occur to a number of important structures associated with the hard tissues, pulp and periodontium. Two very important determinants of control are bur depth and angulation.

This particular skill should be practised from a very early stage. You must ensure that the head of the handpiece and the associated bur are visible at all times to allow you to make an informed judgement about your working depth and orientation. It is also critical that you are aware of the dimensions of the burs you are using; that you have adopted a comfortable and healthy seating position; and that you have employed an effective finger rest.

First steps

Initially these exercises should be carried out:

- On the bench, outside of the mouth
- Within simple ivorine blocks (approximately 15 mm × 15 mm)
- Using the high-speed handpiece
- With a water-cooled, pear-shaped diamond bur

Using a pencil, draw the letter X into the face of your block, leaving a border of around 2 mm. The aim here is to work perpendicular to the flat plane of the ivorine block to create a very simple X-shaped cavity. Your pencil outline should be the guide.

Basic principles – undercut

A 2 mm long pear-shaped bur corresponds to the average thickness of occlusal molar enamel. It is a useful bur with which to practise optimising your undercut (retention form) and cavity form.

Wherever you choose to enter and exit your cavity preparation, you will sacrifice retention form: the full width of the bur is drawn through the block and so that part of the preparation has no undercut.

Once the bur is fully seated, its movement through the block results in a preparation mirroring the cross-sectional shape of the bur – this means that the base of the preparation is wider than the surface, resulting in an undercut preparation.

Clearly, then, the retention form of your preparation is determined not only by the location of your entry and exit points, but by the number of times the bur has been withdrawn from the block. When thinking about your X-shaped preparation, it would seem sensible to use the centre for entry and exit, keeping the bur fully seated as you extend up and back down each of the four arms.

Basic principles – cutting depth

If the bur is *fully seated* and *perpendicular to the surface*, then it will move through the block relatively easily, leaving a smooth cavity floor of uniform depth and optimal undercut.

If the bur becomes seated too deeply, then the stainless steel shank will prevent the bur moving through the block. At this point, the base of the bur will rotate upwards and forwards. In an attempt to regain control, the bur is often then raised until it begins to move through the block once again. This see-sawing action results in a cavity floor of uneven depth with a sub-optimal degree of undercut.

Conversely, if the bur is not fully seated, then the cavity will have little undercut throughout. The opportunity to use the dimensions of the bur to create inherent undercut will have been missed. In order to create undercut thereafter, the bur will need to be used to revisit the lateral cavity walls and the preparation may become excessively wide. When revisiting a preparation, avoid 'resting' the bur on the floor of the cavity – *hold* it at the height at which you want it to cut. This is a little like a hot knife through butter – draw on your desired path rather than letting it cut through the base of the existing preparation indiscriminately. A finger rest is absolutely critical here.

Criteria for exercise

Your preparation should demonstrate the following features:

- Smooth outline form (no jagged or rough edges)
- Accurate preparation (following your prescribed lines)
- Consistent depth (2 mm)
- Undercut throughout the majority of the preparation
- Not excessively wide (no greater than 1.5 mm)

You will notice that if the high-speed handpiece is not running at full speed then:

- The bur will receive insufficient water cooling. As a result, the block and bur will burn, and the diamond coating will be lost.
- The torque will be reduced and the bur is likely to stop within the block, resulting in it binding or fracturing.

Once you have developed enough control, you can move on to other letters involving curves or more elaborate shapes requiring careful consideration of entry and exit points. At this point, you should move towards working on simulator teeth and natural teeth within your phantom head.

Practising with occlusal surfaces

Using a pencil, draw over the major fissures of a molar tooth. This will form the basis for your preparation. The outlines here are very artificial, because ultimately it will be caries that determines where tooth tissue is to be removed. This is just an exercise in handpiece control within the phantom head.

At this time you can begin to think about:

- Maintaining an even depth despite an uneven occlusal contour
- Visibility and planning your entry and exit points
- Maintaining angulation perpendicular to the surface
- Centring your preparation within the fissure
- Gaining access to the preparation with restorative instruments
- Engaging with critical appraisal and peer review

It is also important to begin thinking about unsupported and fragile tissue, especially adjacent to the marginal ridges. In small premolars you may need to extend into the mesial or distal pit and develop a rounded terminus, rather like one end of a dog's bone. This results in a smooth, rounded preparation rather than a thin, forked preparation that is likely to propagate a fracture.

9 Investigating and controlling the carious lesion

Figure 9.1 Carious lesions

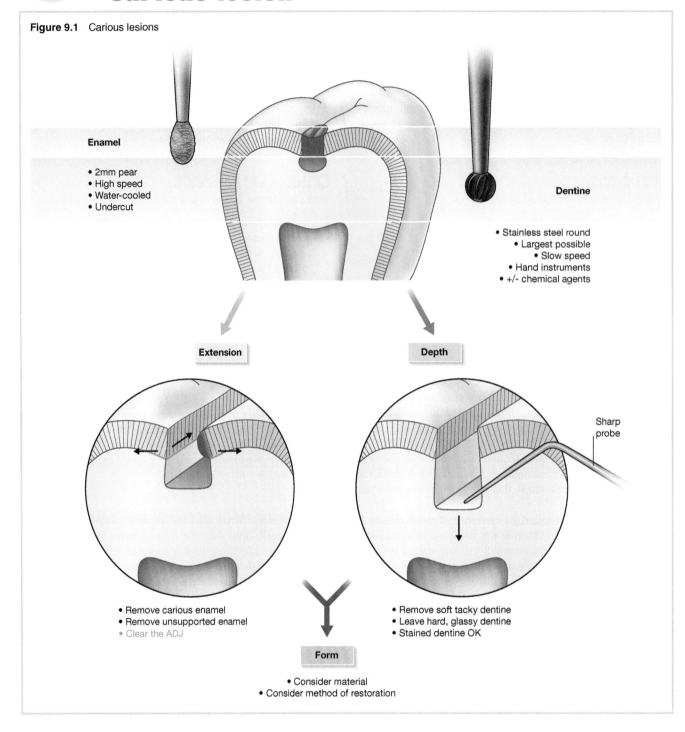

Enamel

- 2mm pear
- High speed
- Water-cooled
- Undercut

Dentine

- Stainless steel round
- Largest possible
- Slow speed
- Hand instruments
- +/- chemical agents

Extension

Depth

Sharp probe

- Remove carious enamel
- Remove unsupported enamel
- Clear the ADJ

- Remove soft tacky dentine
- Leave hard, glassy dentine
- Stained dentine OK

Form

- Consider material
- Consider method of restoration

Pre-Clinical Dental Skills at a Glance, First Edition. James Field. © 2016 by John Wiley & Sons, Ltd. Published 2016 by John Wiley & Sons, Ltd.
Companion website: www.wiley.com/go/field/preclinical-dental-skills

Once the carious process has extended beyond the enamel layer, operative intervention becomes a necessity. Preventive techniques will no longer be able to halt the caries as it progresses through the softer dentine beneath. The true extent of the carious lesion may be hidden clinically by the resilient enamel layer. It is for this reason that the diagnostic process should involve radiographic assessment in addition to the clinical signs and symptoms. If the caries is extensive, then the enamel layer may well have 'cavitated' and collapsed, leaving the wider carious lesion exposed. In either case, the primary aim is to create a preparation that will allow a well-sealing restoration to be placed. Even if the preparation is revisited at a later date for further caries removal, the peripheral seal should prevent further substrates entering and therefore halt the progression of the lesion. More often than not, preparations into dentine will require the use of local anaesthetic to ensure patient comfort.

Basic principles

Regardless of where the lesion exists, it is important to consider the following principles:

- Conservative access
- Efficient removal of tooth tissue
- Ensuring that all carious enamel is removed
- Clearing the amelo-dentinal junction (ADJ)
- Removing any unsupported enamel

Conservative access

Occlusally the extent of your access preparation may vary considerably, depending on whether you are investigating an early enamel lesion (enamel biopsy) or wanting to access frankly carious dentine. In contrast, accessing an interproximal lesion will require a definite preparation through enamel and into dentine, extending at least as low as the contact point. Either way, it is important to plan your access carefully to ensure that tooth tissue is conserved where possible:

- What bur will you use initially?
- How deep will you prepare your initial access?
- How will you monitor your working depth?

Efficient removal of enamel

In order to remove carious and unsupported enamel, it will be necessary to use a diamond-coated bur with water coolant. A 2 mm pear-shaped bur in the high-speed handpiece is the most appropriate choice. The length of the bur corresponds to the average height of occlusal molar enamel, and the wider base creates retention form at the periphery.

Extension

It is important to remove all carious enamel and ensure that the amelo-dentinal junction (ADJ) is cleared. Without a clear ADJ, you will be unable to place a well-sealing restoration. The degree to which the enamel layer is affected will determine the *extent* of your preparation; it may become more extensive if unsupported enamel is removed in preparation for a non-adhesive restoration.

Once the ADJ is cleared, it is then possible to address the central body of the lesion, knowing that a stable, well-sealing restoration can be placed at any point. This may become critical in larger lesions where removal of carious dentine takes you close to the pulp space. You really do not want to be managing a pulpal exposure or even dressing a tooth that has had the pulp space accessed, with carious and unsupported tooth tissue at the margins.

Efficient removal of dentine

Dentine is significantly softer than enamel and as such it cuts very easily with a high-speed diamond bur. If you then consider that carious dentine is softer still, you can understand why when using the high speed there is a real risk of over-preparing your cavity. Once into dentine, you should be using the slow-speed stainless steel burs. These are more effective at discriminating between carious and healthy dentine. It is important to make sure that the following apply:

- The slow-speed handpiece is running in a forward direction.
- You are using the largest possible stainless steel bur.

These factors will ensure that you are removing carious dentine as efficiently as possible. A good finger rest is critical here. Hand instruments such as excavators are available for even more discriminate caries removal. When the dentine is not in proximity to the pulp space, chemo-mechanical caries removal is also possible. This reduces both the vibratory effect of the handpieces and the mechanical effort required with excavators alone.

Depth

Chronic carious lesions may present with dark staining, although this is not in itself a reason to remove the dentine. When assessed with a straight probe, active lesions will present with leathery or tacky surfaces and frankly carious dentine will be softer still. Your preparation should ideally finish on a relatively hard, glassy dentine base regardless of the colour. On occasion, particularly when working close to the pulp space with a risk of exposure, it may be acceptable to leave a slightly tacky layer of dentine, provided that a well-sealing restoration can be placed. Do not be afraid to remove frank active caries.

Form

The form that the final preparation takes will be largely dependent on the extension and depth of the carious lesion. However, it is also important to think about:

- the restorative material in terms of strength in section, resistance to axial loading and retention form;
- maintaining rounded internal line angles to reduce crack propagation and subsequent fracture.

Simulation exercises

If you have access to natural extracted teeth, take the time to examine those that present with intra-coronal restorations. Carefully, using a rounded tapered crown bur, progressively pare back the tooth tissue and identify the restorative interface. Are you able to observe any cracks, fractures or deficiencies? Have there been any noticeable pulpal responses to the operative intervention? Are you able to identify any secondary or tertiary dentine deposition?

10 Posterior approximal preparations

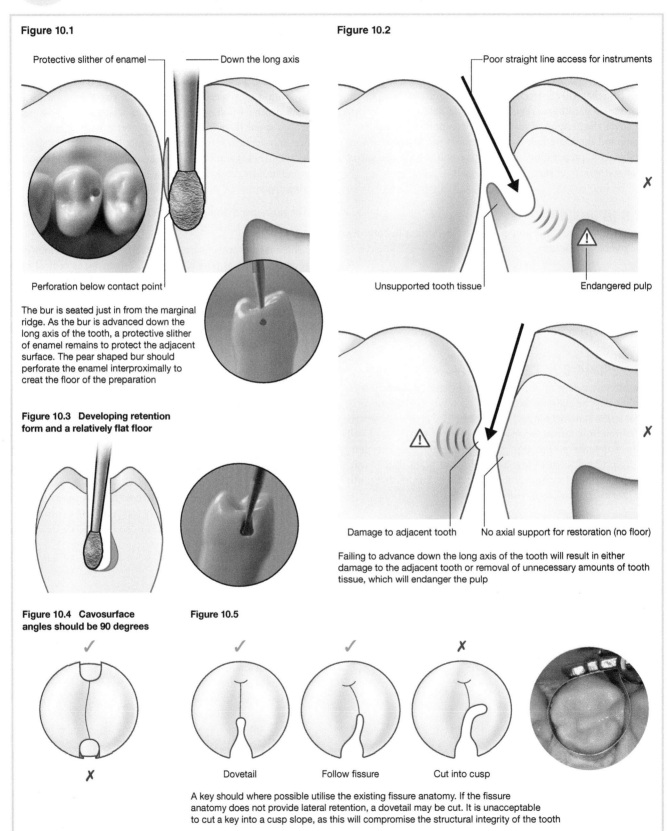

Figure 10.1

Protective slither of enamel — — Down the long axis

Perforation below contact point

The bur is seated just in from the marginal ridge. As the bur is advanced down the long axis of the tooth, a protective slither of enamel remains to protect the adjacent surface. The pear shaped bur should perforate the enamel interproximally to creat the floor of the preparation

Figure 10.3 Developing retention form and a relatively flat floor

Figure 10.4 Cavosurface angles should be 90 degrees

Figure 10.2

— Poor straight line access for instruments

Unsupported tooth tissue   Endangered pulp

Damage to adjacent tooth   No axial support for restoration (no floor)

Failing to advance down the long axis of the tooth will result in either damage to the adjacent tooth or removal of unnecessary amounts of tooth tissue, which will endanger the pulp

Figure 10.5

Dovetail   Follow fissure   Cut into cusp

A key should where possible utilise the existing fissure anatomy. If the fissure anatomy does not provide lateral retention, a dovetail may be cut. It is unacceptable to cut a key into a cusp slope, as this will compromise the structural integrity of the tooth

Pre-Clinical Dental Skills at a Glance, First Edition. James Field. © 2016 by John Wiley & Sons, Ltd. Published 2016 by John Wiley & Sons, Ltd.
Companion website: www.wiley.com/go/field/preclinical-dental-skills

Approximal refers to the surfaces of teeth that contact, or are adjacent to, one another. Although there are clinical signs relating to advanced approximal lesions, lesions remaining in enamel or reaching just past the ADJ are often only noticed on bitewing radiographs. An enamel-only lesion would normally be treated preventively with interproximal cleansing and the use of a fluoride mouthwash with regular review. If the lesion extends into dentine, then operative intervention is necessary. Classically the interproximal carious process begins at the contact point, a poorly accessible area where plaque and other substrates stagnate. A typical posterior approximal preparation, therefore, needs to remove the carious tooth tissue, so the contact point itself must be cleared. This preparation is very technique sensitive and is arguably one of the most difficult techniques at this stage of your skills development. Direct vision of the base of the preparation while instrumenting is unlikely to be possible, and there is real potential to damage the adjacent tooth if the high-speed handpiece is poorly controlled. Most skills courses require you to demonstrate access from the occlusal surface. It is also possible to access from the buccal surface or the mesial or distal pit (as a tunnel preparation). Of course sometimes, where there is no approximating tooth, you may have direct access.

Technique

You must be *very clear* about what you want to achieve here. The aim is to create a preparation that clears the contact point while being as conservative to healthy tooth tissue as possible and without needlessly endangering the health of the pulp. The preparation should be able to receive a restoration that is supported axially and is (unless adhesive) retained in an occlusal and lateral direction. Finally, the preparation should be finished in such a way that it has rounded internal form and no unsupported enamel. The pear-shaped bur should be used for the initial access, followed by a round stainless steel slow-speed bur for any necessary further caries removal. Hand instruments should be used to finish the margins and line angles within the preparation.

Gain access to the caries

A 2 mm pear-shaped bur is most useful for this preparation. Be mindful of *where* on the occlusal surface you are beginning your preparation. You should enter as close to the marginal ridge as possible, while leaving a thin slither of enamel in place to protect the adjacent tooth. You can break this slither away with hand chisels later. Because of the approximal concavity below the contact point, the pear-shaped bur will perforate through to create a window interproximally just below it. The risk of damaging the adjacent tooth at this point is low, assuming that the bur is sited down the *long axis* of the tooth (Figure 10.1).

Resistance and retention form

Once the bur has cleared the contact point, it is possible to introduce resistance and, where necessary, retention form into your preparation. Often removal of the contact area will also remove the actively carious tooth tissue in an early or moderate-sized lesion. However, if the carious lesion is more extensive, it may

be that the removal of tooth tissue from the body of the tooth provides adequate resistance and retention form. It is important to consider this when designing your preparation.

The preparation should primarily allow a restoration to be supported axially, that is, down the long axis of the tooth, while being loaded from the occlusal surface. In order to do this, a non-adhesive restoration such as amalgam should have a relatively flat floor perpendicular to the long axis. A non-adhesive restoration also needs retention form in both an axial and a lateral direction. The base of the preparation can be widened slightly, making use of the dimensions of the pear-shaped bur or even a large stainless steel slow-speed bur. With the former, the handpiece head should be rotated slightly towards the lateral and then medial aspects of the preparation (Figure 10.3). Try not to simply pull the bur in a lateral or medial direction, otherwise the entirety of the preparation will become excessively wide. An occlusal key within the existing fissure pattern can also provide retention axially and laterally. The key should be at least 2 mm deep to ensure that the restoration is strong enough in thin section. Using a pear-shaped bur and accessing from the interproximal area will ensure that you maximise the undercut (and therefore axial retention form). Normally an occlusal key would follow a fissure pattern for around 2 mm. If the fissure pattern is completely straight (and would therefore offer no lateral retention form), it is possible to prepare a small dovetail into the end of the key. It is not acceptable to curve a key into a cusp slope (Figure 10.5).

Common pitfalls

It is very common at this stage to prepare initial access too far onto the occlusal surface, or to allow the bur to deviate from the long axis of the tooth. If the bur deviates towards the body of the tooth, then there is a risk of missing the contact point while endangering the pulp. Furthermore, this error leaves a large lip of dentine towards the base of the preparation, rather than a flat floor. This lip will be too large to manage with hand instruments alone and so it will be necessary to revisit the base of the preparation with the high-speed bur (increasing the risk of damage to the adjacent tooth). If the bur deviates towards the interproximal space, then there is a risk of damaging the adjacent tooth, and failing to obtain a floor to the preparation and any associated axial resistance that this provides (Figure 10.2).

Finishing the margins

The margins should be finished with a chisel to ensure that there is no unsupported enamel. The angle that the cavity margin creates as it meets the outer tooth surface – known as the cavo-surface angle – is around 90 degrees (Figure 10.4). Gingival margin trimmers can be used to bevel the margins of the box and key.

Criteria for critical appraisal

- Removing the contact point
- Rounded internal line angles
- No unsupported enamel
- Not compromising the pulp
- No damage to the adjacent tooth
- Adequate retention and resistance form

11 Anterior approximal preparations

Figure 11.1 Removing contact area leaving protective slither of enamel

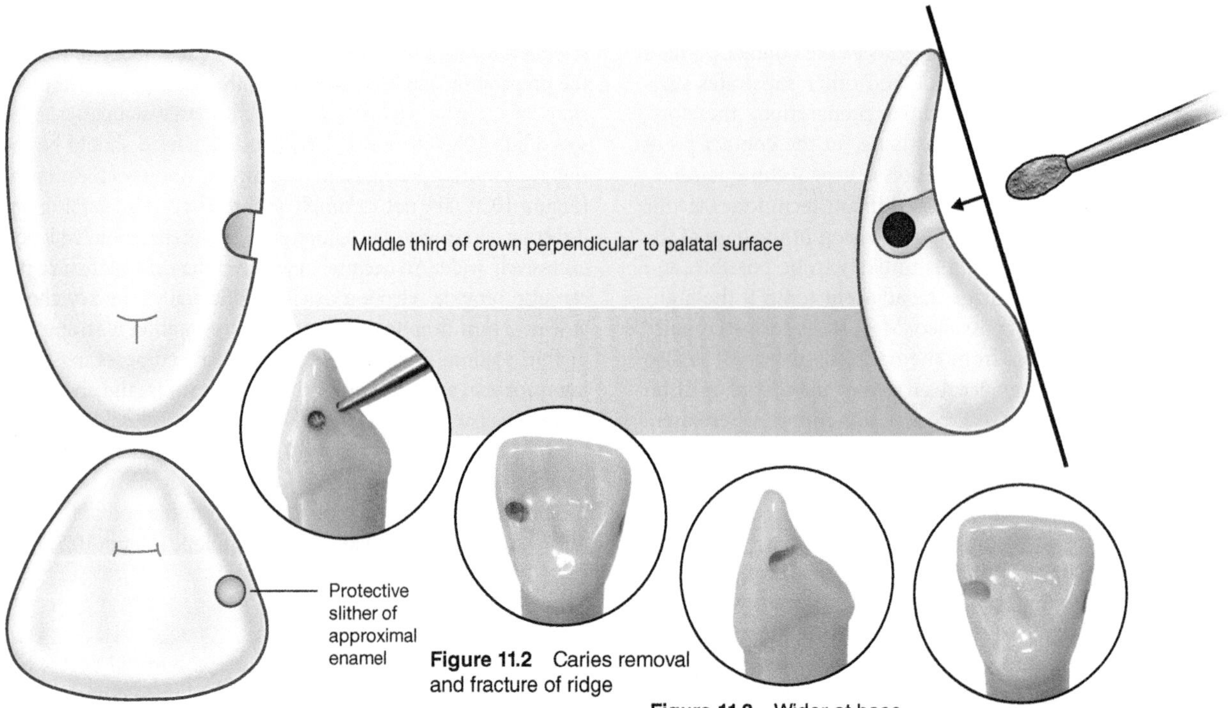

Middle third of crown perpendicular to palatal surface

Protective slither of approximal enamel

Figure 11.2 Caries removal and fracture of ridge

Figure 11.3 Wider at base with minimal palatal access

Figure 11.4 Cavosurface angles 90 degrees with no supported enamel

Figure 11.5 The preparation should be slightly visible from the full labial surface and remain withing the middle third of the crown

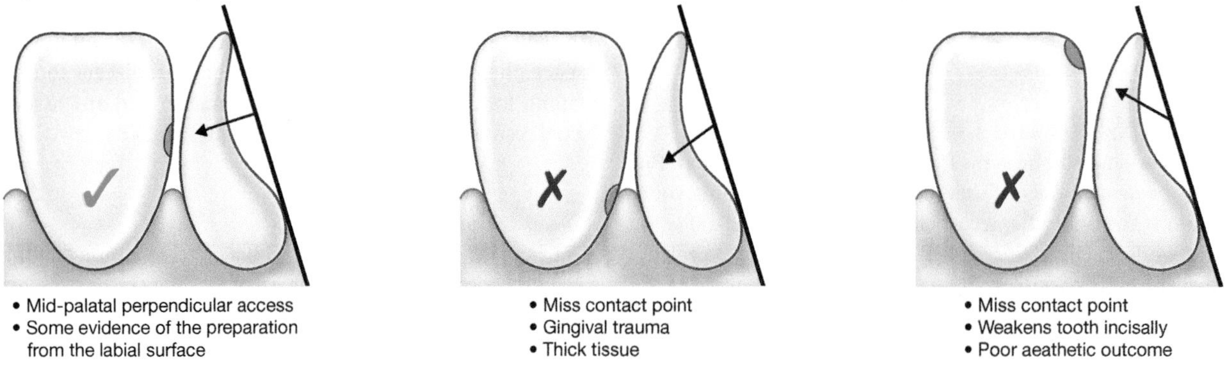

✓
- Mid-palatal perpendicular access
- Some evidence of the preparation from the labial surface

✗
- Miss contact point
- Gingival trauma
- Thick tissue

✗
- Miss contact point
- Weakens tooth incisally
- Poor aeathetic outcome

Pre-Clinical Dental Skills at a Glance, First Edition. James Field. © 2016 by John Wiley & Sons, Ltd. Published 2016 by John Wiley & Sons, Ltd.
Companion website: www.wiley.com/go/field/preclinical-dental-skills

Anterior approximal lesions are often first noticed clinically; even early carious lesions can cast a significant shadow through the relatively thin approximal tissues. Standard bitewing radiographs do not involve the anterior teeth, and dental panoramic radiographs show poor detail, particularly around the midline. Further investigation of anterior lesions may therefore involve periapical films.

The treatment options are comparable to the posterior approximal lesion. An enamel-only lesion would normally be treated preventively with interproximal cleansing and the use of a fluoride mouthwash with regular review. If the lesion extends into dentine, then operative intervention is necessary. Again, the interproximal carious process begins at the contact point, a poorly accessible area where plaque and other substrates stagnate.

This preparation is also technique sensitive, requiring removal of the contact point. Although direct vision of the preparation is more achievable than for posterior preparations, the anterior lesion sits within the aesthetic zone and involves thinner sections of tooth tissue. The depth of the preparation therefore becomes more critical.

Technique

In order to minimise the aesthetic impact, access of small lesions is usually carried out from the palatal or lingual surface (Figure 11.1). Extensive lesions may already have cavitated onto the labial surface, in which case direct access may be possible.

The aim is still to create a preparation that clears the contact point while being as conservative to healthy tooth tissue as possible and without needlessly endangering the health of the pulp. It is most likely that an adhesive composite restoration will be placed into this preparation, so it should be finished in such a way that it has rounded internal form and no unsupported enamel.

The pear-shaped bur should be used for the initial access, followed by a round stainless steel slow-speed bur for any necessary further caries removal. When preparing lower incisors, some clinicians prefer to use a small round diamond bur. It is important to try this technique, but be careful about controlling the bur depth; once the small round head disappears into the tissues, it can be difficult to know how deep you are working. Hand instruments should be used to finish the margins and line angles within the preparation.

Gain access to the caries

Again, be mindful of *where* on the occlusal surface you are beginning your preparation. The initial palatal or lingual access is more difficult than a posterior occlusal surface due to the steep angulation and smooth, flat presentation. Ideally your access should be within the middle third of the crown (in a inciso-apical direction). The bur should be parallel to the palatal or lingual surface.

A 2 mm preparation will in most cases ensure that you have reached the contact point. It is essential to leave a thin slither of enamel in place to protect the adjacent tooth (Figure 11.2). You can break this slither away with hand chisels later. Because of the approximal concavity below the contact point, the pear-shaped bur will perforate through to create a window interproximally just below it (Figure 11.1). The risk of damaging the adjacent tooth at this point is low, assuming that the bur is sited perpendicular to the palatal surface. It is more difficult to gauge the mesio-distal orientation of the bur, but this is offset by the ability to observe the bur directly as it penetrates towards the labial surface. In order to clear the contact point sufficiently, the preparation should be *slightly* visible from the full labial surface (Figure 11.5).

Resistance and retention form

The preparation is most likely to receive an adhesive composite restoration, so there is no need to prepare retention form deliberately. However, there is a need to maintain *minimal palatal access*, while ensuring that the full contact area is removed along with any associated carious tooth tissue. It is therefore recommended that the base of the preparation be widened slightly, making use of the dimensions of the pear-shaped bur or even a large stainless steel slow-speed bur (Figure 11.3). The restoration is also unlikely to be loaded axially (unless it is extensive and involves the incisal edge), so there is no need to develop a flat floor to the base of the preparation.

Common pitfalls

It is very common for this type of preparation to be too conservative and to fail to clear the contact point effectively. There must be evidence of the preparation from the labial surface.

Bur angulation is critical, particularly in relation to the palatal surface. Often the access point is correct, but the bur angulation is poorly controlled and deviates apically or coronally. An apical direction will result in a deep preparation that misses the contact point. In addition to working through a thick layer of tooth tissue, you may also cause gingival trauma. Working too coronally will also result in a preparation that also misses the contact point, but further results in a large amount of unsupported enamel incisally.

Finishing the margins

The margins should be finished with a chisel to ensure that there is no unsupported enamel and that the cavo-surface angles are 90 degrees (Figure 11.4). Gingival margin trimmers can be used to bevel the margins of the preparation.

Criteria for critical appraisal

- Removing the contact point
- Slightly visible from the full labial surface
- Rounded internal line angles
- No unsupported enamel
- Not compromising the pulp
- No damage to the adjacent tooth

Accessing the pulp space

Figure 12.1 Accessing the pulp space

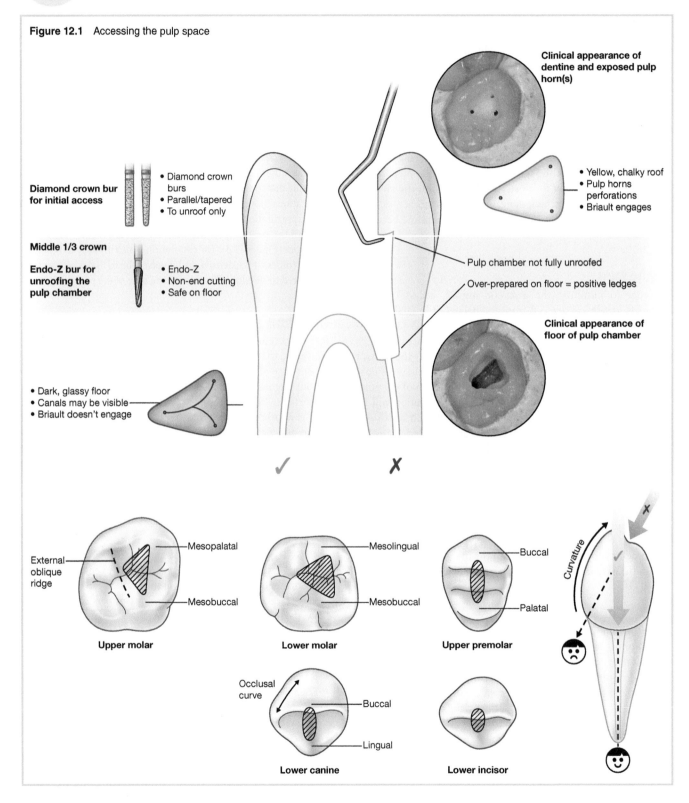

Diamond crown bur for initial access
- Diamond crown burs
- Parallel/tapered
- To unroof only

Middle 1/3 crown

Endo-Z bur for unroofing the pulp chamber
- Endo-Z
- Non-end cutting
- Safe on floor

- Dark, glassy floor
- Canals may be visible
- Briault doesn't engage

Clinical appearance of dentine and exposed pulp horn(s)

- Yellow, chalky roof
- Pulp horns perforations
- Briault engages

Pulp chamber not fully unroofed

Over-prepared on floor = positive ledges

Clinical appearance of floor of pulp chamber

External oblique ridge

Mesopalatal
Mesobuccal

Upper molar

Mesolingual
Mesobuccal

Lower molar

Buccal
Palatal

Upper premolar

Occlusal curve

Buccal
Lingual

Lower canine

Lower incisor

Curvature

Pre-Clinical Dental Skills at a Glance, First Edition. James Field. © 2016 by John Wiley & Sons, Ltd. Published 2016 by John Wiley & Sons, Ltd.
Companion website: www.wiley.com/go/field/preclinical-dental-skills

Entering the pulp space of an intact tooth is one of the most challenging basic skills that you will be required to develop. It is very much a test of your ability to assess tooth angulation and control the handpiece in three dimensions. At this stage, most skills courses will be interested in your ability to locate and fully unroof the pulp chamber only; there is no immediate requirement to delve deeper looking for entrances to root canals, which comes later.

Clinical considerations

Clinically there are a number of things to consider prior to entering the pulp space proper, such as whether root canal treatment is necessary or whether it is possible to remove a small portion of the affected pulp coronally, leaving vital tissue beneath (particularly relevant during a carious exposure). The latter is known as a pulpotomy and contrasts with complete removal of the pulp tissue (pulpectomy). Local anaesthetic is recommended when entering the pulp space of teeth; often some vital pulp tissue remains even though teeth may appear non-responsive to testing. Furthermore, soft tissue anaesthesia makes isolation with the rubber dam clamp more comfortable. It is acceptable to access the pulp space without a rubber dam in order to help maintain the correct orientation of the approach; however, it must be applied before the commencement of root canal treatment to protect the patient and allow the use of otherwise harmful chemical irrigants.

Pulp space anatomy

It is important for you to know the typical anatomy of the pulp space for each tooth type. With this in mind, you will be able to design the shape of your access cavity to ensure optimal and conservative removal of tooth tissue. Excessive removal of tooth tissue coronally weakens the tooth and reduces retention form for a temporary restoration. Excessive tissue removal towards the floor of the pulp chamber increases the risk of perforation. Radiographs can help you estimate the angulation of the tooth and the size and shape of the pulp chamber. It may be that the pulp space has become calcified or sclerosed coronally, necessarily increasing the depth of your access preparation.

Aims

Fully unroofing the pulp chamber is important for several reasons:

- It facilitates total removal of necrotic and infected pulp tissue, which may perpetuate infection or discolour the tooth.
- It creates a cleansable cavity space.
- It creates a smooth preparation free from ledges, which will facilitate instrument use for subsequent root canal treatment.

Technique

Almost without exception, the pulp space is accessed from the occlusal aspect. The angulation of approach is critical, so a relatively long bur should be used to prepare down the long axis of the tooth. A longer bur will also allow you to monitor your working depth. Often finding the pulp space is likened to 'drilling for oil' – a bur is driven into the centre of the tooth until it drops down into the space below. This is a dangerous approach, which can result in aggressive preparations and perforations. In fact, the process of finding the pulp space should be careful and controlled.

I often compare accessing the pulp space to finding Narnia – not only because you should not expect to find it on every occasion, but because many hours can go by while you are trying. Know your anatomy and work at the correct angulation, constantly stopping and checking from all angles. It is extremely tempting at larger depths to 'go fishing' for the pulp space and deviate from the long axis, but this will also undoubtedly result in a perforation. It is better to 'happen upon' the pulp space while remaining within the central body of tooth tissue. If you find yourself working at or beyond 8 mm, it may be time to stop and seek further advice. Clearly, then, it is important to understand the dimensions of the burs that you are using.

Pulp horns will have a fairly close relationship to the cusp anatomy, but initially access can be confined to a more conservative area. As a rule of thumb for posterior teeth, access can be prepared within the tips of the two major cusps and the centre of the tooth (see Figure 12.1). Once the pulp space has been accessed, you can then ensure that the chamber is fully unroofed. It is important to try to preserve important structural characteristics such as oblique ridges on upper molars, as these will afford extra structural durability in an otherwise compromised tooth.

As a rule of thumb:

- Incisors – prepare a triangle with the apex just encompassing the cingulum and the base up to the incisal edge.
- Mandibular incisors and canines – access often involves the incisal edges or tips.
- Canines – prepare a bucco-palatal oval between the incisal edge and the cingulum.
- Premolars – prepare a bucco-palatal oval, up to but not involving each cusp tip.
- Maxillary molars – being careful of the oblique ridge, prepare a triangle between the palatal cusp, mesiobuccal cusp and central pit mesial to the oblique ridge.
- Mandibular molars – prepare a triangle with the apex centrally within the tooth and the base between the mesiobuccal and mesiolingual cusp tips.

A high-speed parallel fissure bur or crown bur is useful for beginning your initial access shape. Continue to advance down the long axis of the tooth, being careful to maintain your access shape. When into dentine (which will appear as a yellow, chalky base beyond 2 mm in depth), stop and check every millimetre or so for pulp horn exposure using a straight probe. Once you have exposed a pulp horn or dropped into the central pulp space, there is no further need for high-speed end-cutting burs. The floor of the pulp chamber should be protected at all costs in order to avoid ledging at canal entrances, or perforations. Instead, the remaining roof should be brushed away using either a high-speed Endo-Z bur (which is non-end-cutting) or a large slow-speed stainless steel bur. With the latter, the roof should be removed on the outward stroke only. A Briault probe should be used to check that the walls are ledge free and the chamber is fully unroofed.

Common pitfalls

Initially you might confuse exposed pulp horns for the entrances to root canals. Verify the depth at which you are working, the colour of the base of your preparation, and whether a Briault probe can engage under the remaining roof.

If you have set your teeth up in plaster, clear the cemento-enamel junction (CEJ) to expose the full crown – you will be able to assess the long axis more effectively. Do not be distracted by the plane of the occlusal surface, especially on anterior teeth and lower first premolars.

13 Direct posterior restorations

Figure 13.1 Direct posterior restorations in amalgam

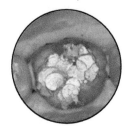

- Pack into deepest part first
- Ensure well condensed
- Overpack then curve back

Overpack amalgam

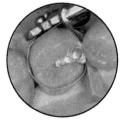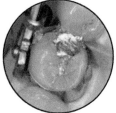

Pack into the deepest part first and then overpack

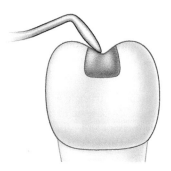

Occlusal

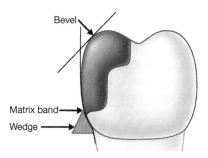

Bevel

Matrix band

Wedge

Approximal

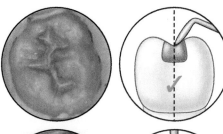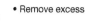

- Remove excess
- Use half Hollenbach to rest on natural tooth tissue wherever possible to avoid under/over-carving

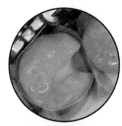

- Ensure matrix adaptation at base (check with probe)

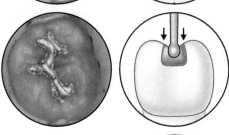

- Avoid burnishing material to the sides, resulting in thin unsupported ledge of material

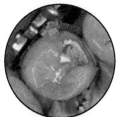

- Note position and height of marginal, ridge and prescribe bevel

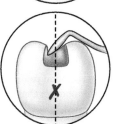

- Avoid advancing half hollenbach past central fissure

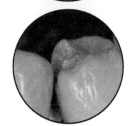

- Care when removing matrix if using amalgam to avoid marginal ridge fracture
- Check for flash and that floss can be passed through the contact

Occlusal carving using the half Hollenbach

Approximal carving using the half Hollenbach

Pre-Clinical Dental Skills at a Glance, First Edition. James Field. © 2016 by John Wiley & Sons, Ltd. Published 2016 by John Wiley & Sons, Ltd.
Companion website: www.wiley.com/go/field/preclinical-dental-skills

A direct restoration relates to material that is placed into a preparation or cavity in an unset form. The material then undergoes a setting reaction either by chemical cure, light cure or both. Because material can be adapted to the tooth before setting, the term 'plastic' restoration is often used. The same principles of material and instrument handling apply to all direct restorations.

Occlusal restorations are often considered to be the most straightforward. Approximal restorations involve the replacement of a mesial or distal surface; on these occasions the occlusal element is often overlooked, resulting in a poorly adapted restoration. The pictorial examples in this chapter relate to the use of amalgam, as this is considered to be the most technique-sensitive material with respect to working time and irretrievability (relating to under-filling, voids or fractures). Although it is necessary to ensure that composite is incrementally placed, well-adapted and fully cured, there is scope to make indefinite further modifications and repairs. An important element to consider when placing restorations is the occlusal relationship with the opposing arch, although this is not within the scope of this chapter.

Material choice

The choice of restorative material should have been considered during preparation of the cavity, and would typically be either amalgam or composite resin. Critical to the success of an amalgam restoration is the requirement for adequate retention form. The amalgam will not be chemically bonded to the tooth tissue and so it is important to think about how it will be mechanically retained and remain durable when loaded. The preparation should be as conservative as possible, while maintaining a minimum thickness of material (1.5 mm) in order to avoid fracture. Unsupported enamel should be removed, as this will fracture away in function. It is possible to chemically bond amalgam restorations into place using either a very small amount of cement lute (glass ionomer) or a resin-based lute. In the former it is important to ensure that cement remains at the base of the preparation and does not extrude to the periphery; this would prevent the amalgam from forming a corrosive seal with the tooth tissue.

A composite restoration will require effective moisture control, but will provide far superior aesthetics. There is also less need to consider retention form, as the composite will be chemically adhered to a layer of unfilled resin, which in turn is retained through micromechanical retention to the tooth tissue. The composite resin actively splints the tooth and so unsupported tissue is less of a concern. Glass ionomer is not an ideal choice in this situation due to its inferior compressive and tensile strength.

Instrumentation for amalgam

It is extremely important to ensure that your amalgam will be contained while you condense it, either by four walls of natural tooth tissue or by using a matrix band to replace one or more walls. The matrix should be secured with a wedge and have good adaptation at the base. Ideally this should be checked with a probe. In the skills lab you will most likely be using an alloy with a working time of between 7 and 8 minutes. You must therefore pack the amalgam effectively and efficiently. Start at the deepest part of the preparation, using the largest possible instrument to condense each increment. You should use a reasonable amount of force and your fingers may well ache after the first few occasions you condense the material. A mercury-rich layer may appear on the surface as a shiny film, and this should be scraped away periodically. It is a good idea to over-pack with amalgam: while excess can be easily carved back within the setting time, it is much more difficult to mix and pack further increments. If you are restoring an approximal surface, pay close attention to the height of the marginal ridge – use a straight probe to bevel the approximal surface and then reduce the height of the ridge before attempting to remove the matrix band and carve the occlusal surface. The band should be removed carefully, avoiding a levering action that may dislodge the relatively brittle marginal ridge. It is possible to hold a condenser against the ridge while removing the band to protect its integrity. At this point, it is worthwhile checking that floss can be passed through the approximal surface, and any flash (thin film of material overlaying cavity margins) is removed.

The half Hollenbach is a particularly useful instrument. The leaf-shaped tips facilitate the contouring and restoration of occlusal anatomy. Where possible, the instrument should be continually resting on natural tooth tissue. This ensures that no flash remains at the margins of the restoration, but also that the restoration is not over-carved. It is used through a paring action (the edges of the leaves should be cutting, not the tip directly). A good finger rest should be employed as the instrument is worked down the cusp slopes until the tip rests in the central fissure. Take care not to extend the tip past the centre, otherwise you will carve away material from the opposite cusp slope.

Your restoration may sometimes look a little flat at the base. This can occur for two main reasons:

- The restoration may have been under-filled or over-carved.
- The restoration may have been under-carved. In this situation, the instrument must be taken further down the cusp slopes until the tip rests centrally within a fissure.

While excavators and burnishers can be useful for developing mesial and distal pits within the restoration, care should be taken to ensure that material is not inadvertently dragged from the margin of the restoration. Often burnishers can result in a relatively flat anatomy accompanied by a thin lip of unsupported material at the periphery. This will fracture away in function, leaving a failed margin.

Instrumentation for composite

Composite requires a dry field. The material should be packed and cured in increments to minimise the effects of polymerisation shrinkage. It is not possible to 'condense' composite, but the material is thixotropic, so it can be encouraged to adapt to the cavity by 'puddling' the surface with the condenser at a rate of about six times per second. The maximum depth of cure should be noted, otherwise the composite can be left with an uncured 'soggy' bottom. Composite affords you the luxury of being able to make further additions, contouring and polishing without being limited by time. A range of discs, strips, interproximal files and finishing burs are available to ensure that the restoration is well finished.

Common mistakes

The most frequent problems are that matrices are poorly adapted, amalgam is not condensed effectively, and restorations are under-carved. Do not be afraid to use the natural tooth tissue to support and guide the half Hollenbach.

14 Replacing a cusp with a direct restoration

Figure 14.1 Replacing a cusp with a direct restoration

Amalgam

Composite

- Retain mechanically with slots in dentine at opposite sides of the preparation or chemically using traditional or resin cements

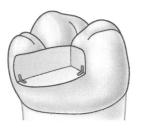

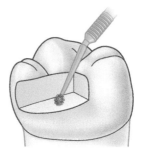

- Acid-etched, primed and bonded with appropriate moisture control

- Overpack and then remove the band - take care not to fracture the ridge

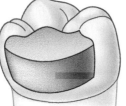
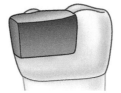
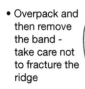

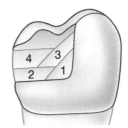

- Incrementally pack composite if the depth of cure is less than 2 mm and the shrinkage is greater than about 1.5%

- Final layer leaves cusp bevel

- Carve the cusp bevel

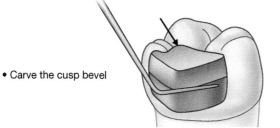

- Check appropriate ridge height. If high, polish back with high-speed diamond burs. Refine the cusp bevel with polishing discs

- Choose marginal ridge height

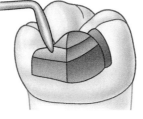
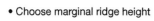

- Look from all angles to assess morphology
- Carve occlusal pits, fissures and the mid-buccal groove

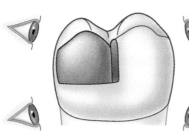

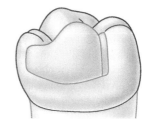

- Occlusal pits, fissures and the mid-buccal groove can be refined using high speed composite burs

- Check for final contour and flash before finishing with polishing paste

Pre-Clinical Dental Skills at a Glance, First Edition. James Field. © 2016 by John Wiley & Sons, Ltd. Published 2016 by John Wiley & Sons, Ltd.
Companion website: www.wiley.com/go/field/preclinical-dental-skills

When relatively large amounts of coronal tooth tissue are missing, a decision must be made about whether to restore the tooth definitively with a direct restoration (amalgam or composite) or a laboratory-made indirect restoration (composite, ceramic or metal). This chapter considers the direct restoration of a missing cusp with a plastic restoration. Although in future there may be a requirement to move away from mercury-based materials, there is still considerable educational value in learning to restore with amalgam while in the skills laboratory. As such, this chapter considers both amalgam and mono-phase composite techniques.

Preparation

While practising to restore a large cusp in the skills lab, it is worthwhile initially cutting an approximal box with an occlusal key. This ensures that the preparation at least clears the contact point and has sufficient occlusal extension. The key can then be extended peripherally to remove the relevant cusp and the associated smooth-surface groove. At this point it is important to consider how the direct restoration will be retained. For amalgam, the restoration will require mechanical retention in the form of slots, or chemical bonding with cements. Composite bonding relies on micromechanical retention of a resin layer, and this system along with silane-coupling agents can also be used to bond amalgam restorations into place. If required, retention slots should be prepared on contralateral dentine walls, approximately 1.5 mm from the lateral border, using a small round slow-speed bur. The slots should be no more than 2 mm in length and 1 mm in width, ideally at the junction between the floor and axial wall of the preparation. A contralateral slot will afford both proximal and occlusal retention form.

Matrices

Regardless of which material is to be placed, a well-fitting matrix band must be adapted to the tooth. Ideally this should be secured with a wedge. If using a Siqveland system, the positioning of the retainer is very important when replacing the buccal wall of a tooth – it should sit passively in the sulcus with the toggle engaged at the base. Many operators avoid this position when restoring a buccal cusp, because the confluence of the matrix sits adjacent to the intended restoration. However, placing the retainer on the medial side often means that it catches on the anterior teeth and twists the matrix band. Although the effect is not immediately obvious, it makes restoration quite difficult, as the band buckles out mesiobuccally and pulls away from the intended position of the marginal ridge. The Tofflemire system allows the use of an 'angled' retainer that overcomes this problem. In any case, once the band is tightened, a rounded instrument such as a probe or Mortenson's condenser should be used to burnish the matrix up to the contact point. Take care not to over-tighten the band, which will tend to narrow the cusp; once the band is seated, place an interproximal wedge before tightening the retainer just enough to secure the base of the box. If the confluence of the bands does sit adjacent to the restoration, then this area should simply be contoured once the band has been removed. Ensure that the band is high enough to restore up to cusp height.

Technique for amalgam

Amalgam needs to be condensed effectively and efficiently in order to give yourself time to carve and finish the restoration. It is very important to have a sequence of events in your mind. Over-pack the amalgam initially, ensuring that you have plenty of height from which to fashion the replacement cusp.

1 Remove gross excess overlying remaining tooth tissue with the half Hollenbach and then choose the position of your cusp tip. Look carefully at the existing cusps – cusp tips are rarely positioned at the periphery of the restoration. This is due to the cusp bevel.

2 Carefully remove the matrix band in an occlusal direction only rather than using a rocking motion – the latter will often fracture away material interproximally.

3 Work down from your cusp tip in four directions using the half Hollenbach carver:
  • Carve a cusp bevel, which should effectively draw your cusp tip in from the lateral border.
  • Choose the height of your marginal ridge – use the contralateral cusp and adjacent marginal ridge as a guide.
  • From the marginal ridge, begin to carve your fissure pattern, ensuring that you excavate a mesial or distal pit. The ridge should be the dam, the pit should be the lake bed and the fissures are the river – without a pit, the fissures will be too shallow and the ridge will lack definition.
  • Finally, check your contour from *all angles* and re-create a smooth-surface groove to give the cusp more definition.

4 Pass floss through the contact and check for flash at the margins.

Technique for composite

Most standard composites will need to be incrementally packed to ensure a full depth of cure and to minimise polymerisation shrinkage. If this is the case, then once the preparation is etched, primed and bonded, the composite should be built up in small increments from the deepest part first. Unlike amalgam, composite cannot easily be carved back once it has been command set. It is preferable to fashion the intended anatomy into the composite *before* it is cured, with minor adjustments made through polishing thereafter. Once the floor of the preparation is covered, it is possible to build a peripheral wall that reaches the intended height of the marginal ridge. At this point the matrix can be removed, and the restoration can be completed as a class 1 occlusal restoration. It is necessary to pay attention to the same occlusal features, but there is less emphasis on time. Point 3 above should still be considered, but most of these features will already have been prescribed while placing the increments. Finishing the external contour is arguably more difficult with a tooth-coloured material; it is easy to leave flash or even significantly larger amounts of composite overlying unbonded enamel, which will suffer from fracture and/or microleakage. Be wary of overheating the tooth with polishing discs, and be mindful that even fine diamond high-speed polishing burs will cut into natural tooth tissue relatively easily. It is very important to check for interproximal excess and ledges, which can normally be corrected using strips, Eva files (Kavo®) or judicious use of a tapered finishing bur.

15 Placing cervical restorations

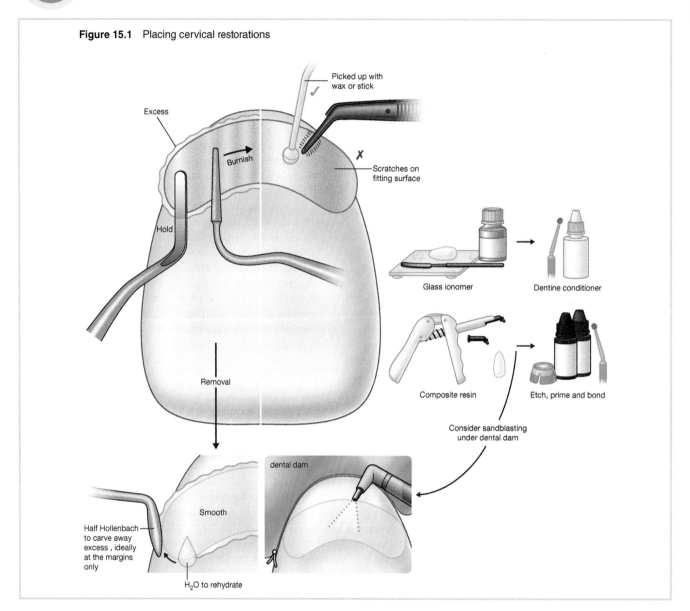

Figure 15.1 Placing cervical restorations

Excess

Burnish

Picked up with wax or stick ✓

✗ Scratches on fitting surface

Hold

Removal

Glass ionomer → Dentine conditioner

Composite resin → Etch, prime and bond

Consider sandblasting under dental dam

Smooth

Half Hollenbach to carve away excess , ideally at the margins only

H₂O to rehydrate

dental dam

Pre-Clinical Dental Skills at a Glance, First Edition. James Field. © 2016 by John Wiley & Sons, Ltd. Published 2016 by John Wiley & Sons, Ltd.
Companion website: www.wiley.com/go/field/preclinical-dental-skills

Cervical restorations are relatively easy to place: more often than not they are situated on the buccal aspect where there is good access and direct vision. The real challenge is placing a restoration that has longevity – and the cervical area is arguably the most difficult in this respect. It is subject to a fairly unique group of processes and forces, the most significant of which are:

- Caries
- Abrasion, most likely from tooth brushing
- Abfraction from flexural movements of the tooth on loading
- Erosion from intrinsic or extrinsic sources

It is important to understand the underlying pathology, because the aetiology of the lesion is also likely to be responsible for the loss of the restoration.

When deciding which material to restore with, it is important to consider:

- The proximity of the lesion to the gingival margin
- The ability to control moisture in the area
- Aesthetics
- Caries risk

Glass ionomer

Glass ionomer is often used because it is relatively moisture tolerant, is quick and easy to place, and forms a chemical bond to the tooth tissue. While this is true, placing glass ionomer cements freehand will result in a relatively rough restoration that will readily pick up a biofilm; this results in the accumulation of staining and mature plaque. Glass ionomers have the added benefit of leaching fluoride into the immediate vicinity, but this is unlikely to be effective at preventing further carious tissue loss if significant plaque deposits are allowed to accumulate. Glass ionomers can be polished but only after their full-phase set, otherwise there is a significant risk of desiccation and mechanical/aesthetic failure.

Arguably, the best way to ensure the smooth finish of a cement restoration is to use a matrix. A standard cellulose matrix strip is inappropriate, because it will buckle when adapted to the curved cervical region. An aluminium cervical matrix is preferred, which can be burnished over the lesion using a flat plastic or a Mortenson's condenser. Care should be exercised when handling the matrices, and you should try not to pick up a matrix with anything metal (like tweezers or forceps) as the beaks will scratch the polished surface. The scratches will then be transferred into the surface of the final restoration, or may cause the cement to lift out with the matrix. It is possible to use a small bead of carding wax on the end of a hand instrument to pick up the matrix. It is also possible to buy little wax-ended sticks that look like cotton buds – but don't put them into your ears!

Burnish the matrix over the empty lesion and set it aside, paying attention to the orientation with which you seated it. It is important to condition the dentine using a polyacrylic acid prior to placing the cement onto dentine. The key here is to ensure that the final restoration requires as little modification as possible, and ideally no instrumentation over the main body of the restoration. This should ensure a perfectly smooth finish. It can be difficult initially to gauge how much cement is required, but it is often less than you think. Clearly voids are undesirable, but at the same time you want to avoid lots of excess escaping from the matrix. Once the cement is in place, seat the matrix firmly and hold it in place on both sides using your hand instruments. Keep a small amount aside to monitor the setting reaction.

Once the material has become brittle, you are able to lift off the matrix. Often a probe or half Hollenbach tip is very useful here. You will undoubtedly notice a small amount of excess around the periphery and this should be carved away. It is important once the matrix is removed that the glass ionomer does not desiccate – instrumentation will cause this to happen very readily and you will observe the cement becoming chalky in appearance. If this does occur, simply dab a damp cotton pellet over the surface to rehydrate it. In some circumstances, poor adaptation of the matrix or gross overfilling means that almost the entire body of the lesion needs to be carved back. A decision should be made at this point about whether a new restoration should be placed or if the final roughness is acceptable. Ideally, a thin layer of protective varnish should then be placed, although most modern glass ionomer cements do not require this.

Composite resin

Where moisture is controllable and the lesion sits above the gingival margin, it may be possible to use a composite resin restoration. It can be difficult to isolate the lesion under rubber dam without using a floss ligature technique or butterfly clamp, and sometimes it is best just to employ good aspiration, cotton rolls and dry tips – even retraction cord (under local anaesthetic). The lesion should be etched, primed and bonded as normal, and the restoration can be placed and polished in the usual way. Clear plastic matrices are available, but these are unable to be burnished to adapt closely to the tooth's anatomy. Take care that flash does not encroach on the biological tissues, especially into the buccal sulcus.

Repeated restoration loss

Cervical restorations have a reputation for failing relatively soon, and this can be due to any of the processes mentioned above working in isolation or in combination. It might be necessary to consider preparing some form of mechanical retention, especially if the lesion is rather shallow and dished out. However, the cervical area sits within relatively close proximity to the pulp. Preparing into this region would also further weaken the tooth.

In cases of repeated loss or where highly sclerotic dentine is present, it may be that micromechanical forms of retention such as etching need to be supplemented with sandblasting. This will undoubtedly require the placement of dental dam, at least for the sandblasting procedure.

16 Restoring incisors

Figure 16.1 Restoring incisors

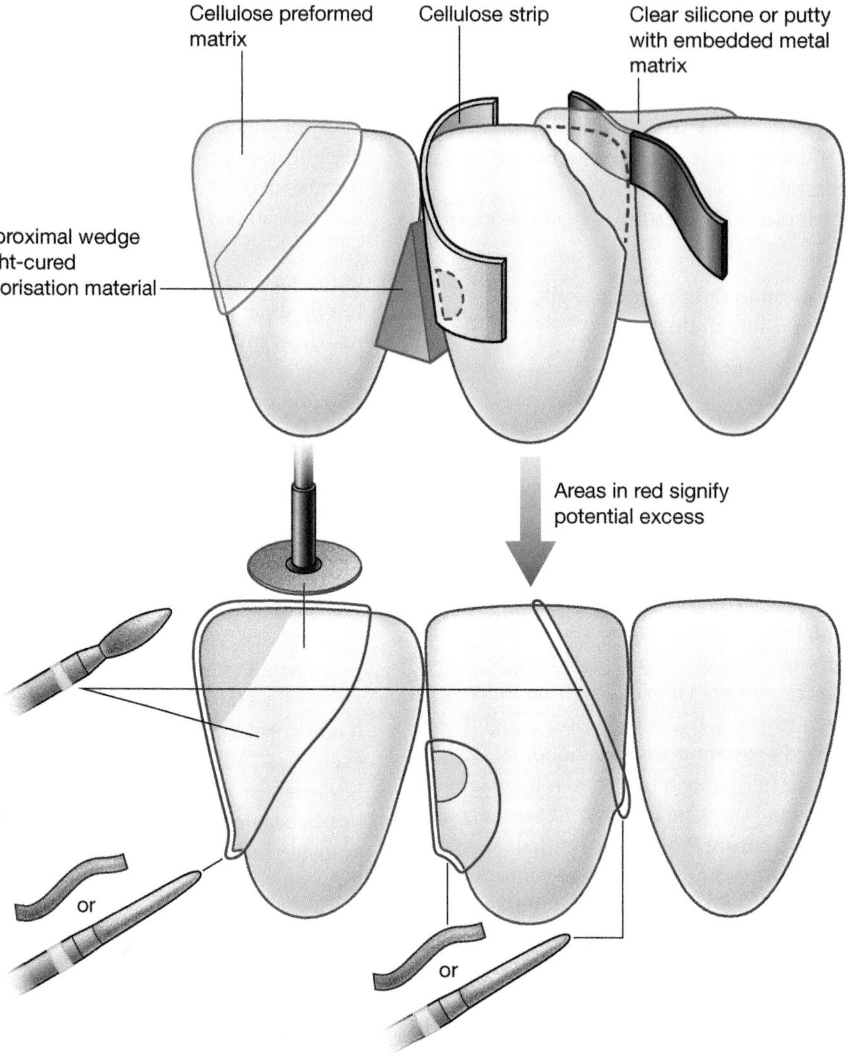
Cellulose preformed matrix
Cellulose strip
Clear silicone or putty with embedded metal matrix
Interproximal wedge or light-cured temporisation material
Areas in red signify potential excess
or
or

Pre-Clinical Dental Skills at a Glance, First Edition. James Field. © 2016 by John Wiley & Sons, Ltd. Published 2016 by John Wiley & Sons, Ltd.
Companion website: www.wiley.com/go/field/preclinical-dental-skills

The basic restoration of incisors may be required following an approximal preparation, or loss of part of an incisal corner or edge. Often skills courses will require you to combine the two, giving you a more holistic opportunity to use composite placement and polishing techniques. If you are asked to prepare an incisor for restoration within the skills laboratory, it is a good idea to begin with an approximal preparation (see Chapter 11) and then to extend your preparation towards the incisal edge, to involve at least one third of the tooth width. Placement of the rubber dam should be routine for these types of restoration, although it may be that you need to use a split dam technique in order to be able to restore up to the approximal tooth surface. In order to optimise the aesthetic outcome, an appropriate shade should be selected; it is best to do this before isolating and drying the preparation. Composite tends to stick to stainless steel instruments and where possible gold-coated or Teflon-coated instruments are recommended. The material should be 'puddled' into place rather than packed, to allow it to flow appropriately and minimise voids.

Achieving an optimal bond

It is important to consider how you will achieve an optimal bond to tooth tissue. For preparations with a clear enamel periphery, this will not be an issue. Sometimes it is appropriate to bevel the enamel margins in order to increase the area for enamel bonding. Often in cases where teeth are heavily worn and sclerosed, it is appropriate to consider sandblasting as an adjunct.

Approximal restoration

The approach described in Chapter 11 details preparation from the palatal or lingual aspect in order to minimise the aesthetic impact. Restoration follows similar principles, with placement of a matrix that forms a smooth labial surface at the base, and incremental placement of composite from the palatal/lingual aspect. A clean smooth matrix is essential and (as when placing a posterior approximal restoration) good marginal adaptation is key. More often than not a clear cellulose matrix is required to allow light curing of the composite – this can be held in place with an interproximal wedge. Alternatively, light-cured temporary restorative material such as Fermit or Systemp (both from Ivoclar Vivadent) can be used in order to better contour the interproximal area and hold the matrix in place. This can be picked out later once the restoration has been cured. The matrix needs to be pulled tight across the labial surface in order to reduce the escape of excess material. It should be cured before incrementally packing and curing the remainder towards the lingual/palatal surface.

Involving the incisal edge

This type of restoration is much more demanding, given that you are required to manage more than three surfaces – approximal, labial, lingual/palatal and incisal. It is possible to restore all but the incisal edge first using a cellulose strip, but care must be taken to contour the incisal third appropriately thereafter, otherwise the resulting restoration requires considerable adjustment. Several other methods are available to help restore the intended anatomy:

- A *preformed cellulose crown* that can be cut back to restore the intended tooth structure. This method is quick, but can result in an overly bulky restoration with lots of excess, especially interproximally.
- A *putty or clear silicone index* that has been fabricated on a waxed-up model. This method is accurate and allows the restoration to be built up in discrete layers, allowing the use of dual-phase composites that comprise separate enamel and dentine shades. Care should still be taken around the interproximal area, although it is possible to embed an interproximal strip into the matrix to separate adjacent teeth. The matrix is usually seated lingually/palatally and built up towards the labial aspect. This can be almost impossible if the teeth require lingual/palatal restoration with no associated labial tooth tissue loss – once the matrix is seated you cannot gain access to place the composite or cure it.
- A *clear plastic index* fabricated using a vacuum or pressure over a waxed-up model. Again this is accurate, and care should be taken around the interproximal area. Adjacent teeth can be effectively separated by wrapping with polytetrafluoroethylene (PTFE) tape. Often this technique is favoured as it facilitates light curing from all angles during placement.

Polishing and checking

It is very easy to leave excess interproximally and on each smooth surface (see areas outlined in red in Figure 16.1). This should be managed with convex high-speed diamond finishing burs lingually/palatally, slow-speed discs labially, and with interproximal strips. When using polishing discs, ensure that you work through the full range. The coarsest discs (often darker in colour) will readily change the form of the restoration, while the smoother discs will only polish. Bear in mind that coarse discs can cause considerable damage to the soft tissues and even to natural tooth tissue both directly and by overheating; use them in short bursts while polishing. For more significant interproximal ledges that cellulose strips are unable to remove, once again consider metal strips, Eva files (Kavo) or judicious use of a tapered finishing bur.

Repairing existing restorations

From time to time it is necessary to repair an existing composite or ceramic restoration. Unless the restoration is removed, there is no available enamel and dentine to which to bond. Old composite is compromised as there will be little remaining monomer to bond to, and ceramics/porcelain will not form a chemical bond to the new resin. In these situations it is preferable to etch the surface (to clean it) and then to sandblast (with a silane coupling agent if appropriate) in order to obtain micro-mechanical retention.

Common problems

Take care not to pull an approximal strip too tightly within the coronal third, otherwise the contact point will be poor and the approximal surface will be too rounded. Look from all angles not just the labial, including down from the incisal edge. Finally, double and triple check for flash outside the extent of your original preparation.

17 Periodontal instrumentation

Figure 17.1 Periodontal instrumentation

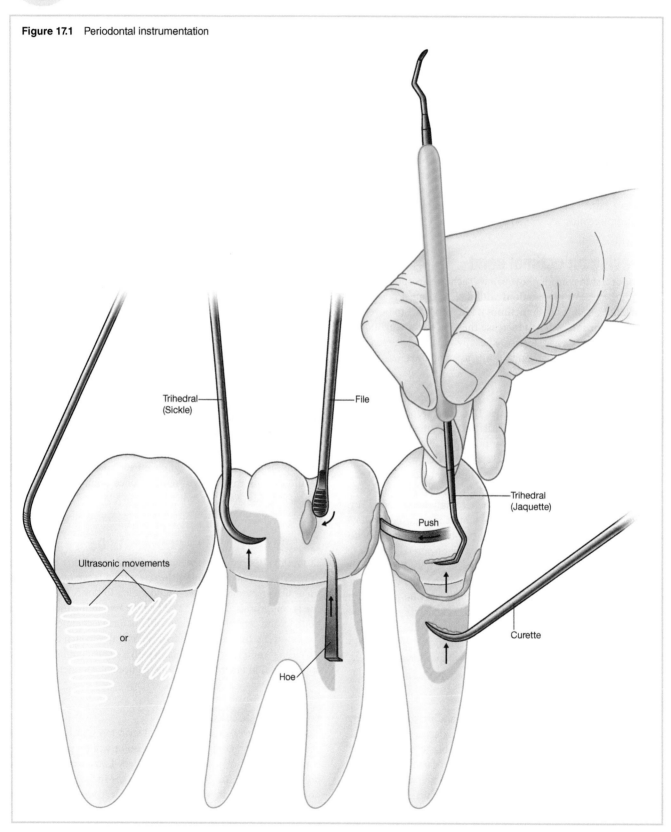

Trihedral (Sickle)

File

Trihedral (Jaquette)

Push

Ultrasonic movements

or

Hoe

Curette

Despite our patients' efforts to maintain adequate oral hygiene, more often than not it is necessary to do the following as a professional:

• Remove calculus deposits from the coronal and gingival aspects of the teeth.
• Remove calculus and necrotic cementum from below the gingival margin and the root surface.
• Disrupt the sub-gingival biofilm.

The aim here is to use the instruments in such a way that the calculus and cementum are effectively removed without damaging the root surface. Often local anaesthetic is required for effective sub-gingival cleaning or if the patient has particularly sensitive teeth.

Hand and ultrasonic instruments both have the potential to cause harm to the hard and soft tissues of the mouth and so should be handled in a controlled way. Table 17.1 outlines the basic range of instrument types, with diagrammatical representations in Figure 17.1.

Before beginning instrumentation, it is a good idea to explore the hard surfaces using a ball-ended probe such as the World Health Organisation probe. This will allow the tactile detection of sub-gingival calculus and help familiarise you with the sub-gingival root anatomy.

Hand instrumentation

You should employ a modified pen grasp, whereby your index finger and thumb are primarily used to hold the instrument. The middle finger rests on the shank to guide the working end and feel vibrations. The ring finger acts as a finger rest, while the little finger is free to float upwards like when drinking tea (scaling is perhaps the most dignified form of tooth cleaning!). The dental mirror can be used for indirect vision/illumination and soft tissue retraction. Take care with the working ends of the hand instruments, as they can easily lacerate the gingivae or sulcal tissues if the tip is not fully engaged on the curved tooth or root surfaces.

It is important to remember that hand instrument strokes are relatively tiny movements, often only a few millimetres at a time:

• *Hand–forearm motion activation*
  Rotating the wrist and arm so that the thumb and forefinger rest in an uppermost position – likened to turning a door knob.
• *Digital motion activation*
  Pulling the thumb, index and middle fingers towards the palm of the hand. Here the hand and the arm do not rotate and this technique is often used where milder forces are required.

Figure 17.1 outlines the intended locations and modes of use for each periodontal instrument.

Ultrasonic instrumentation

Ultrasonic instruments should be held in much the same way as hand instruments. However, it is important to ensure that the tip is never applied directly to the root surface, otherwise this can gouge defects into the tooth. The full working length of the instrument tip should be held flat against the tooth surface in order to encourage hard tissue deposits to become dislodged. Water coolant should be used to prevent overheating and effectively irrigate the area, flushing debris into the oral cavity. It is for this reason that high-volume aspiration is essential during ultrasonic use. Furthermore, the ultrasonic tips have 360-degree activity and so it is important that tooth contact is maintained at all times.

It is also important to test the intended movement or path of the ultrasonic tip prior to activation, as tactile feedback can be altered once the tip is vibrating. The tip should be used in a sweeping action either horizontally or diagonally across the root surface from bottom to top. Normally, ultrasonic tips are activated at low or medium power rather than high power, the latter having the potential to damage the tooth surface considerably.

Table 17.1 Periodontal instruments

	Instrument	Intended location	Mode of action	
Hand instruments	Chisel/push scaler	Supra-gingival Interproximally on anterior teeth	Push stroke through interproximal contact while maintaining contact with tooth surface. Needs sufficient interproximal space and care with gingival tissues	
	Trihedral scaler	Supra and sub-gingival	Adapt the leading third of the cutting edge to tooth surface below calculus deposit. Draw up proximal labial or lingual smooth surface	
	Hoe	Sub-gingival Root surfaces	Pull action parallel to the long axis of the tooth. Must be fully engaged	
	File	Calculus in concave surfaces or tenacious smooth calculus	Requires a strong finger rest while engaging the file edge like an excavator	
	Curette	Sub-gingival Universal or site specific	Terminus has a one-sided cutting edge used with a pull action up the long axis of the tooth	
Ultra sonic	Flat	Supra-gingival Lingual aspects of anterior teeth	360° sweeping action to disrupt the biofilm Practice the movement before activating the tip Diagonal or horizontal sweeps	Medium power flat against the tooth surface
	Rounded	Sub-gingival if accessible Anterior and posterior		Low power Axis of instrument adjacent to tooth surface
	Probe	Sub-gingival Anterior and posterior		Tapping for calculus removal

Moisture control and dental dam

Figure 18.1 Moisture control and dental dam

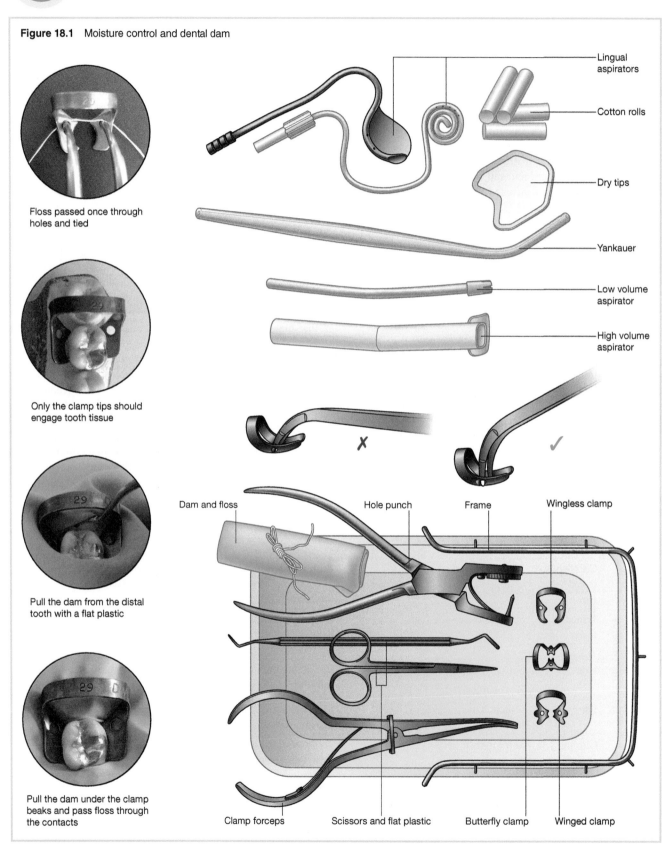

Floss passed once through holes and tied

Only the clamp tips should engage tooth tissue

Pull the dam from the distal tooth with a flat plastic

Pull the dam under the clamp beaks and pass floss through the contacts

Lingual aspirators

Cotton rolls

Dry tips

Yankauer

Low volume aspirator

High volume aspirator

Dam and floss

Hole punch

Frame

Wingless clamp

Clamp forceps

Scissors and flat plastic

Butterfly clamp

Winged clamp

Pre-Clinical Dental Skills at a Glance, First Edition. James Field. © 2016 by John Wiley & Sons, Ltd. Published 2016 by John Wiley & Sons, Ltd.
Companion website: www.wiley.com/go/field/preclinical-dental-skills

Often diagnostic procedures and restorative methods are moisture sensitive, so it is important to be able to keep specific operative areas dry. The most common examples of this are when carrying out a dental examination or when a composite resin restoration needs to be placed. There are also occasions when the mouth in general is excessively moist – this can be due to patient factors (excessive pooling saliva) or operator factors (use of water-cooled instruments and the 3:1 syringe).

Standard aids

The most routine forms of moisture control comprise the use of cotton rolls (in the adjacent sulcus) and aspiration. A range of aspirators are available (see Figure 18.1) and a couple can even be held in place by the patient. Dry tips® (Mölnlycke Health Care) are extremely useful in capturing the saliva produced from the parotid gland, and should be placed adjacent to the upper first molar on the buccal mucosa (matt side down, arrow pointing distally); they can hold up to 30 times their own weight in saliva while remaining flexible enough to move with the soft tissues.

Dental dam

On occasion, further isolation is required. This may relate to moisture control, but it may also be in order to protect the soft tissues from chemical (endodontic irrigants, acid-pumice techniques, bleaching) or abrasive (sandblasting) materials. Dental dam acts rather like a raincoat that is stretched over an operative area and onto a frame. Sometimes the dam loops over the patient's ears with elastic. The area of concern is then isolated from the rest of the mouth.

Dental dam is also provided to improve:

- patient comfort
- airway protection
- visibility
- soft tissue retraction

Although the components of a dental dam kit may differ between surgeries, the main items are shown in Figure 18.1. Many surgeries now use latex-free dam and so the term 'rubber dam' is falling out of favour.

Dam clamps

Clamps are available in a range of shapes and sizes from several manufacturers. The two main posterior clamp types are winged and wingless (see Figure 18.1). Winged clamps allow the assembly of the clamp, dam and frame outside of the mouth. Wingless clamps require the placement of the clamp onto the tooth first, before applying the dam and frame. The latter is often preferable because:

- It is less intimidating for the patient to have a clamp placed first and then dam stretched over it afterwards.
- There is less chance of clamping the wrong tooth.
- There is an opportunity adequately to check the fit and stability of the clamp prior to placement of the dam.

It is imperative that a clamp is chosen so that the four tips (or beaks) of the clamp engage hard tooth tissue. If the clamp is too large, then the rounded body of the clamp arms will engage tooth tissue and the following will occur:

- The clamp will rock and increase the chances of clamp fracture or displacement.
- The clamp tips will traumatise the interproximal soft tissues.

Dam clamps can and do break from time to time. Most often this happens across the bridge. If your clamp looks dull or has an altered finish across the bridge, then discard it and use another. In order to minimise the risk of aspiration, a piece of floss should be passed once through each clamp hole before being tied. Do not wrap floss recurrently around the bridge, as this serves to increase the distance between the two sides of the clamp should fracture occur.

Other clamp types available include:

- Butterfly clamps – high-winged clamps that allow placement over relatively tall and narrow teeth such as incisors and sometimes canines.
- Root surface clamps – relatively aggressive tips for use where little or no coronal undercut is present.
- Plastic clamps – reusable clamps with abrasive-coated tips to aid in retention.

Dental dam placement

Figure 18.1 shows strategic points in the placement process for isolation of a single tooth:

- Select an appropriate wingless clamp.
- Pass floss through the holes and tie together at a length of about 10 cm.
- Place the clamp onto the tooth, taking care to engage only hard tissue. If the clamp rocks, it is probably too large. Ensure that the forceps tips are not tilted in the holes when trying to disengage.
- Once the clamp is stable, punch your hole into the dam, stretch the dam wide and pull it over the bridge of the clamp and the tooth.
- At this point the dam will often be caught on the tooth below the bridge – use a flat plastic to ease it forward into the interproximal space. The dam should immediately sit more appropriately.
- Pull floss through the contacts and push the dam over the clamp beaks.
- At this point it is possible to lift the clamp and re-seat it to ensure full adaptation around the cervical portion of the tooth.

Contraindications and alternatives

Dam is not advised for patients who have problems breathing through the nose, or patients who are unable to understand the rationale for dam use (or tolerate it). Often the dam needs to be split to cover several teeth, for example when contact points have to be restored. This, along with alternatives to using a clamp, is mentioned in Further reading.

19 Records for treatment planning

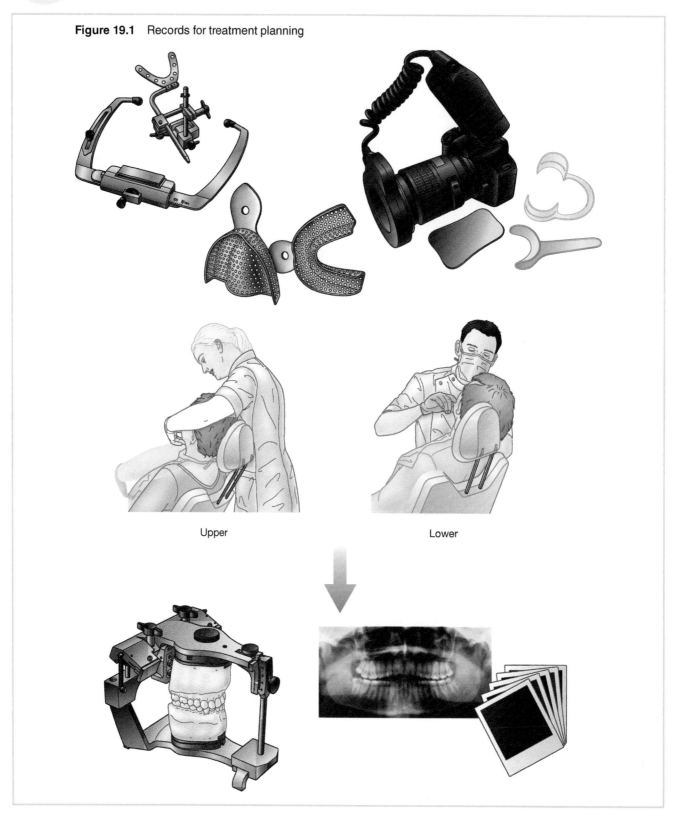

Figure 19.1 Records for treatment planning

Upper

Lower

Pre-Clinical Dental Skills at a Glance, First Edition. James Field. © 2016 by John Wiley & Sons, Ltd. Published 2016 by John Wiley & Sons, Ltd.
Companion website: www.wiley.com/go/field/preclinical-dental-skills

Following a comprehensive history and examination (including radiographs where appropriate), a treatment plan should be devised. Most of the time this will not require any further records. However, on occasion it is necessary to obtain the following:

- Impressions for study models of both arches
- Photographs
- An inter-occlusal record (registration)
- A record of how the maxillary arch relates to the condylar axis (facebow transfer)

These records allow the patient (along with their paper records and radiographs) to be studied and discussed away from the clinic. It may be that a multidisciplinary or team approach is required, that a diagnostic procedure needs to be carried out, or that records may need to be taken over time for monitoring purposes. It is very important to obtain written consent before taking any records.

Study models

Study models should aim to record fully any standing teeth and any edentulous areas. The sulcus should be recorded in its entirety and the impression should be free from air blows and voids. There is no need for a high degree of detail at this stage, but the casts should at least be accurate and trimmed neatly.

Most stock trays will record a full arch, but on occasion you may need to modify the tray either by trimming, expanding or moulding. Few cases require a special closer-fitting tray to be constructed at this stage in order to record the necessary information. In any case, the tray should have retentive features for the impression material and it is always a good idea to use tray adhesive as well. Once the patient is comfortable and has been provided with protective equipment, you should try the trays in the mouth to ensure that the size is correct. Operator position plays a very important role when taking impressions. For an upper arch you should be positioned behind the patient, with your back straight and forearms below your elbows. For a lower arch you should be positioned in front of the patient with a straight back and the full arch in direct view. Do not be afraid to adjust the dental chair to ensure that the patient is at the correct height. It is often easier to stand for these procedures.

Two things that are particularly difficult for students at this stage are:

- Rotating the tray into the mouth. This requires the patient to be relaxed and for you to be controlling the soft tissues with your non-dominant hand.
- Keeping hold of the soft tissues and retracting the lip once the tray is in the mouth and being seated.

Air blows are a common problem, which can be reduced by drying the teeth and pre-loading the alginate into inaccessible areas prior to seating the tray. If taken in alginate, the impressions should ideally be wrapped in damp gauze and cast up the same day.

Inter-occlusal record

Often known as a bite, this record is required in order to relate the upper and lower casts to one another. It is important to think about whether there are enough tooth contacts for your record to be stable (ideally at least tripod contacts), or whether you need to request some wax blocks to provide support in the edentulous areas. You can use putty or compound if the record needs to be done immediately, but wax blocks are usually extended around lingual or palatal aspects and so provide greater stability and ultimately accuracy. A silicone material is preferred over waxes, but care should be taken over the increased accuracy that this provides; often the silicone records more occlusal detail than the alginate and so the registration record does not seat fully onto the cast. If this does happen, trim the fissures away with a scalpel.

Articulation

The way in which the upper and lower casts move in relation to one another (articulate) is primarily determined by the positions of the standing teeth. An average value articulator makes assumptions about the width of the condylar axis, the distance of the maxillary teeth from the condylar axis and the angle at which teeth guide over one another. It is important to think about how this might affect the way in which laboratory work is constructed or planned. For any cases where the existing relationship of the dentition is to be lost – such as increasing the occlusal vertical dimension (opening up the articulator) or altering the existing tooth contacts by extracting, preparing or moving teeth – a patient-specific record of how the maxillary arch relates to the condylar axis is required. This is known as a facebow transfer.

Photos

Most clinicians will use a digital SLR camera, as this allows manipulation of a number of photographic parameters. The main problem with intra-oral photography is a lack of light; however, a standard flash can be very harsh and unidirectional, reflecting off the teeth and soft tissues. A ring flash provides a more measured delivery of light in a more uniform way, reducing flare. The amount of light can also be controlled through the time for which the shutter is open (time value, T) and the distance over which the shutter opens (aperture value, A). There is a fairly complicated interplay between these variables – a larger aperture value means a smaller shutter size. This lets in less light that is more parallel in nature (and so near and far objects are both in focus). The aperture needs to remain open for longer, which increases the risk of blurring. Conversely, a smaller aperture value means a larger shutter opening – this lets in more light, but the light is less parallel and so fewer objects are in focus. It is really important to try the camera away from the clinic to see how the parameters interact. As a rule of thumb, for intra-oral shots I would set a T value of 1/60 and an A value of 12–16; for portrait shots, an A value of about 8.

For shade matching, consider including a piece of white card (for setting white balance) and a labelled shade tab adjacent to the dentition.

Sources of information for each record are suggested in Further reading.

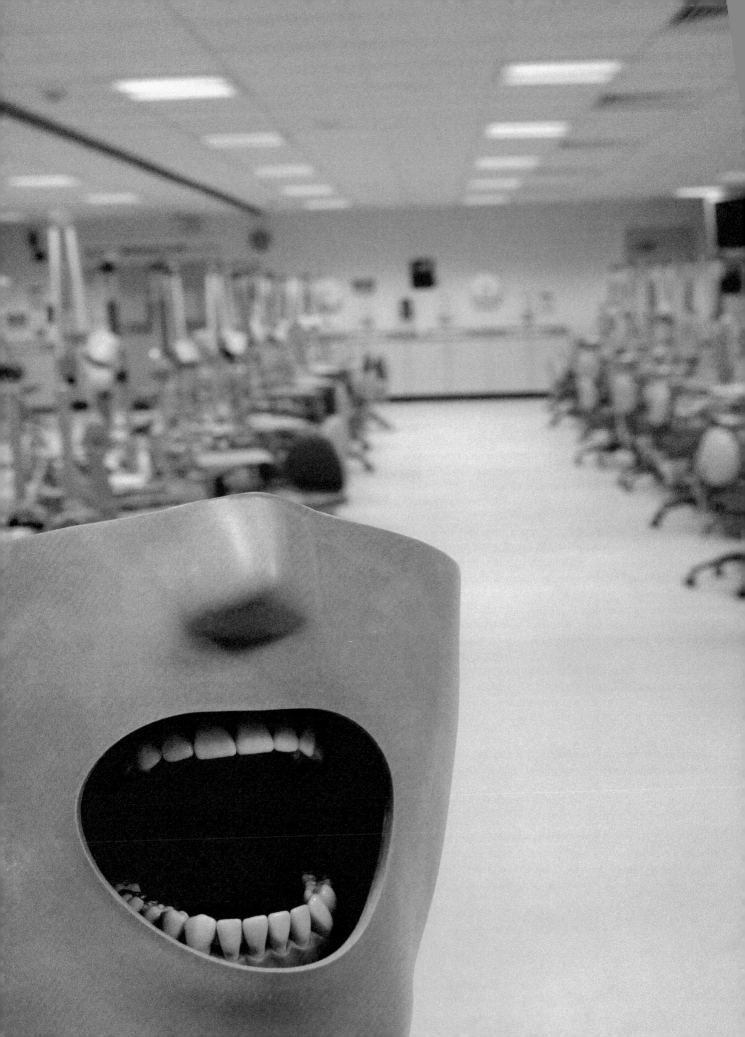

Core clinical skills

Part 3

Chapters

20 Controlling cross-infection

Figure 20.1 Five minutes of clinical activity

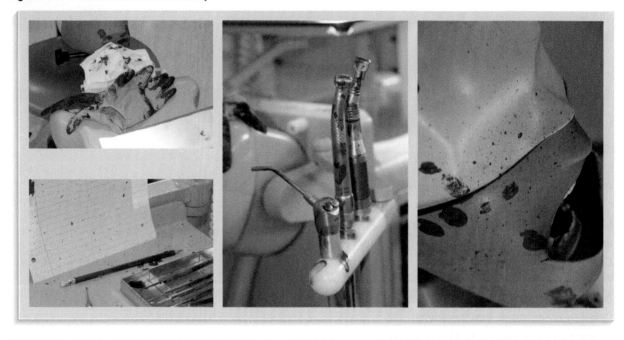

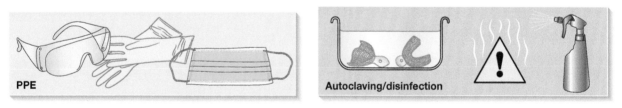

Barriers

Figure 20.2 PPE, zoning, autoclaving/disinfection and handwashing

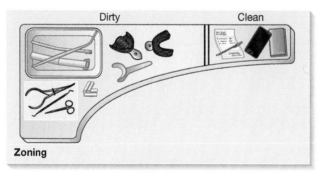

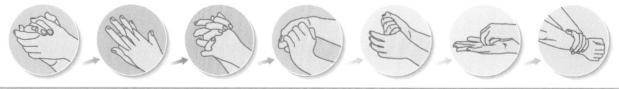

Handwashing
Aycliffe technique

Pre-Clinical Dental Skills at a Glance, First Edition. James Field. © 2016 by John Wiley & Sons, Ltd. Published 2016 by John Wiley & Sons, Ltd.
Companion website: www.wiley.com/go/field/preclinical-dental-skills

When taking a comprehensive medical history you should ask about infectious diseases such as hepatitis, HIV, tuberculosis and herpes. However, your patients are under no obligation to disclose their full medical history and so to ensure safe practice you should treat all patients as an infection risk. This is known as using 'universal precautions'. Diseases can be transmitted through contact with broken skin, saliva, tissue exudate, secretions and blood; most respiratory diseases are transmitted by aerosol. It is important to make sure that suitable barriers are in place to prevent the transmission of infection. These include:

- Effective immunisation
- Using personal protective equipment
- Zoning and reducing risk
- Hand hygiene
- Disinfection and sterilisation

Effective immunisation

In order to work safely within the clinical environment, you need to provide evidence of your vaccination status. This is usually coordinated by your local Occupational Health department. Evidence of hepatitis B, tuberculosis and rubella vaccinations will be requested, alongside routine immunisation against tetanus, polio and diphtheria.

Personal protective equipment

Gloves, masks and eye protection are essential in order to prevent contact and aerosol transmission of microorganisms. The aerosol cloud produced while using the air rotor handpiece is significant and so it is also critical that your operative space is 'zoned' appropriately and that objects within the operative zone are able to be suitably disinfected. Gloves and masks should not be reused.

Zoning and reducing risk

Ensure that you designate a 'dirty' zone within your surgery. Keep non-clinical items such as personal belongings, patient notes and other paperwork well away from your dirty zone. Be aware that the air rotor aerosol will reach over 60 cm from the patient's mouth. You can further reduce the risk of aerosol transmission by using high-volume aspiration. The use of sharps containers will help to avoid unnecessary needlestick injuries, and single-use items will help to break the chain of infection. All staff should be trained to adhere to local protocols and accidents should be logged.

Alongside a local dress policy, you may also be required to work 'bare below the elbow' in order to reduce the risk of cross-infection further. Most of the time a single plain wedding band is acceptable, but you should remove other rings and bracelets.

Hand hygiene

You should wash your hands in any of the following five scenarios:

- Before patient contact
- Before an aseptic technique
- After exposure to bodily fluid
- After contact with a patient
- After contact with the patient's surroundings

A suitable hand hygiene technique will ensure:

- Palm-to-palm contact
- Cleaning of the backs of hands and fingers
- Interlacing of the fingers
- Rubbing of the thumbs and wrists

Hands should be dried with paper towels. Air dryers should not be used in clinical areas as they may spread airborne bacteria. Alcohol-based hand gels are often available at access points to clinical areas, as they can be applied quickly without access to water. However, they are not effective in removing dirt and should only be used if your hands are visibly clean. Patients should also be encouraged to adhere to the hand hygiene policy, as this is equally important in the prevention and control of infection.

Disinfection and sterilisation

Disinfection removes disease-causing organisms but not spores, while sterilisation kills or removes all organisms including spores. The government's Health Technical Memoranda (HTM) provide guidance on decontamination procedures that should be employed within a healthcare setting. They clearly define the roles and responsibilities of a range of key officers with responsibility for aspects of decontamination.

Disinfection is used to treat surfaces, laboratory work prior to transport to the laboratory and instruments that cannot be autoclaved. It commonly involves:

- Alcohols (often as a gel)
- Aldehydes (often glutaraldehyde as a hard-surface cleaner or immersion solution)
- Biguanides (often chlorhexidine as a scrub or solution)
- Halogens (often hypochlorite as an immersion solution)

It is important to ensure that the surgery is completely disinfected after each patient encounter; this includes all surfaces, handles, handpiece connections and controls. All elements of the dental chair, light and spittoon should also be disinfected. Sterilisation is used to treat instruments that are to be reused, and necessarily involves:

- Cleaning – manual or ultrasonic
- Packaging – trays or individual wrapping
- Sterilisation – steam, hot air or chemicals
- Aseptic storage

Sterilisation is most often carried out using steam. The recommended temperature range is 134–138 degrees Celsius at a pressure of 30 psi; this should be held for at least 3 minutes.

21 Communicating and recording information

Figure 21.1 Communicating and recording information

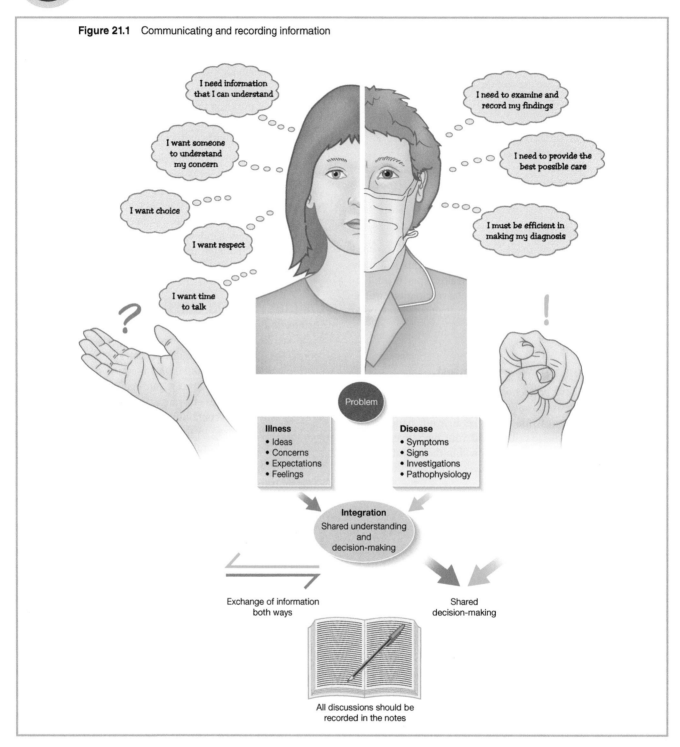

You might wonder why you need to learn about communication; at this stage, you are probably able to articulate yourself pretty well in most situations. Nonetheless, communication is the keystone to a trusting relationship with both patients and the wider dental team, and it deserves special attention within this context. The way in which you choose to interact within your clinical community will depend on the task in hand and the sensitivity of the interaction; this is underpinned by a degree of emotional intelligence and (because it necessarily involves understanding the people with whom you are communicating) critical reflection.

A model for patient communication

As a dental care professional, your primary responsibility is to act in your patients' best interests. In order to understand their problems and complaints, you need to listen very carefully to what they have to say. As a clinician, you also have a responsibility to treat patients in a timely and resourceful way. Often it can seem like a challenge to marry the two together, especially if your patient is nervous or has difficulty recalling information in a logical or coherent manner. Your initial contact with the patient is arguably the most important, often requiring you to negotiate an examination, formulate a diagnosis and agree a contract of care.

Illness vs disease

Healthcare professionals tend to communicate and document information in a very scientific way: measuring sizes, recording facts, determining sequences of events, and looking for causes and effects. This is known as the 'disease framework'. However, patients often speak and think in the language of the 'lived world', based on relationships, causes, personal meanings, myths and metaphors. This is known as the 'illness framework'.

The Calgary–Cambridge framework for communication provides a useful structure for your patient consultation and helps you to account for the different motivators mentioned above. Key to this framework is that the patient feels that you are actively listening to them. It will allow you investigate their Ideas about diagnosis and treatment, any Concerns about the proposed treatment plan, and finally their Expectations for what will be achieved (ICE). The framework comprises the following steps:

- Initiating the session
- Gathering information
- Building the relationship
- Giving explanations
- Shared decision making and planning
- Closing the session

Initiating the session

Greet your patient and introduce yourself and your role. Obtain consent for the consultation and ensure that your patient is comfortable. Demonstrate respect and interest, while identifying the reasons for the consultation using open questions; listen attentively to the responses without interrupting. Screen for further problems and negotiate an agenda, taking both your and your patient's needs into account.

Gathering information

Encourage your patient to tell their story and express their feelings. It is a good idea to use open and closed questions flexibly to facilitate information gathering. It is important to establish dates and a sequence of events. Take the time to explore your patient's ideas, concerns and expectations as well as how the problem affects their life.

Building the relationship

Listen attentively to your patient and facilitate their responses verbally (silence, repetition, paraphrasing, interpretation) and non-verbally (eye contact, facial expression, posture, position). Make notes in a way that does not interfere with your dialogue or rapport. You should demonstrate confidence, yet at the same time be empathic, supportive and sensitive. Share your thinking, explain the rationale for your questions, and seek permission for physical examinations.

Giving explanations

Provide information in manageable chunks, remembering that your patient may have no prior knowledge of their condition or available treatment options. You must check for understanding and ask what other information would be helpful. Use explicit signposting during the conversation so that the patient can keep track of what is being discussed. Your language should be concise and easily understood, avoiding or explaining jargon. Where possible, use visual aids to convey information.

Shared decision making and planning

Try to relate your explanations to the patient's illness framework and provide opportunities for your patient to contribute to the discussion. It is important here to pick up verbal and non-verbal cues and to gauge your patient's reactions and feelings. Again, share your own thinking and offer choices; this will help you to negotiate a mutually acceptable plan.

Closing the session

Towards the end of the assessment, take the time to do some forward planning. When will the next appointment be and for what? Should your patient expect any communication and when? Try to foresee and explain any unexpected outcomes and how your patient should seek help in the meantime. Finally, summarise the session and provide an opportunity for final questions and clarification.

Making a record

The patient record is a legal document. As such, you are obliged to keep it up to date. It should be written contemporaneously (at that appointment) and accurately. If the records are paper based, they should be legible and written in a permanent ink, usually black. When you sign the notes, you should ideally record your designation, GDC number (when qualified) and the date and time. Mistakes should be crossed out and initialled, although earlier entries should not be altered. It is worth remembering that any healthcare professional involved with your patient's care is entitled to request a copy of the patient's notes, regardless of where they are based. Other interested parties may include the police, a solicitor or other individual acting on the patient's behalf, or indeed patients themselves.

22 Giving and receiving feedback

Figure 22.1 Giving and receiving feedback

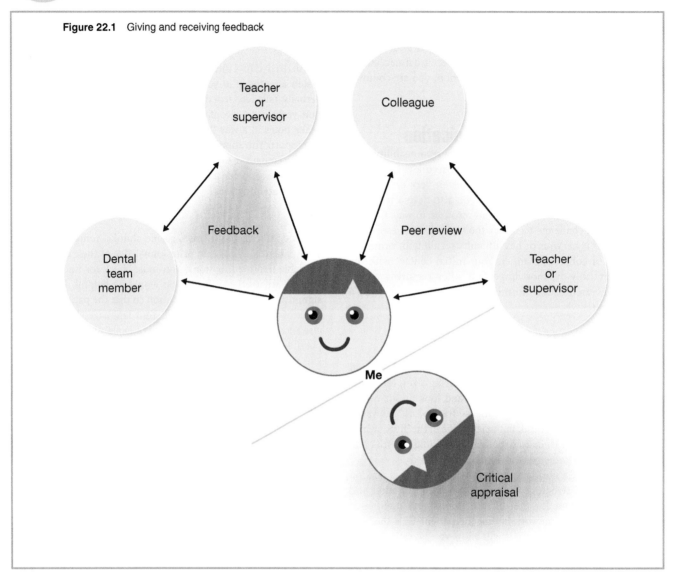

Pre-Clinical Dental Skills at a Glance, First Edition. James Field. © 2016 by John Wiley & Sons, Ltd. Published 2016 by John Wiley & Sons, Ltd.
Companion website: www.wiley.com/go/field/preclinical-dental-skills

The term 'feedback' is used rather ubiquitously and so there is a need to understand it in the context of both higher education *and* working as a healthcare professional.

Feedback within higher education

Higher education should be a challenging yet supportive environment in which you are able to take risks and develop as a curious, independent and confident learner. Feedback plays a very important part in this process. It will relate to some or all of the following:

• A report of your performance both in terms of grade boundaries and in relation to the wider cohort
• Detailing specific areas of good and poor performance
• A description of how to improve
• The opportunity for you to comment on the resources and facilities that are available to you as a learner

Importantly, feedback on your work should not simply comprise 'the answers'. It should be a dynamic and engaging, two-way process involving dialogue between you as a student and your teachers.

Feedback as a healthcare professional

Feedback is important to the ongoing development of learners in healthcare settings. Many clinical situations involve the integration of knowledge, skills and behaviours in complex and often stressful situations. Feedback is central to developing learner competence and confidence at all stages of a medical career.

Within the clinical environment, feedback can be sought from a number of sources:

• Clinical teacher or supervisor
• Dental nurse or other dental care professional
• Colleagues or peers
• Patients

Critical appraisal and peer review

Evaluating your own work is known as critical appraisal. In higher education, nurturing this skill in tandem with reflective practice will help you to develop the capacity to evaluate critically your own and others' performance, to self-monitor and to move towards professional autonomy. Evaluating the work and practice of others is known as peer review.

In order to engage with these processes effectively, it is important for you to have a comprehensive understanding of the task in hand. Within a skills lab, you may often be working to a set of criteria, from which you can benchmark your own and others' progress. Furthermore, peer review is not merely about 'marking someone else's work'; it should be a dynamic process forming a reflective dialogue around your techniques, successes and difficulties. As dental care professionals in primary care, there is potential for us to become relatively isolated from our peers. Alongside continual professional development courses, peer review is a valuable way of catching up with how others are working and sharing good practice.

Receiving clinical feedback

As students or trainees, regular feedback should be provided regarding your knowledge base, clinical work and professional conduct. The aim of this feedback is to help you improve the standard of care you provide to your patients, and to work effectively within the dental team. In order for feedback to be effective, it should be timely (often a dialogue should happen at the time, or at least on the same day). Feedback should also be an open and honest process – you should feel comfortable communicating with your assessors and colleagues and encourage all forms of feedback. When students or trainees do not receive feedback positively, this can inhibit teachers or supervisors from giving regular face-to-face feedback.

Occasionally you may receive comments that seem less than positive, or even that you feel embarrassed or ashamed about. In these situations it is important to do the following:

• Ensure that you have discussed the matter fully with your assessor and that you understand the rationale for their comments.
• Listen carefully to what they are saying and ask for the comments to be repeated if you did not hear them clearly.
• Assume that the feedback is constructive until proven otherwise.
• Ask for examples if you feel that statements are unsupported and ask for suggestions of ways in which you might improve.
• Accept the comments positively rather than being dismissive about them, and thank the assessor for their feedback.
• Set aside some time to reflect critically on the comments and how they make you feel.
• Identify any learning points from the encounter. What might you do differently next time? How might you prepare better for this situation if it occurs again?
• Look to resolve the matter by recording the encounter in a reflective log or portfolio and moving forward in a positive way.

Remember that as a student/trainee you must be accepting of the fact that things can (and do) go wrong. Importantly, you must make the most of each learning experience in order to improve the quality of the care you provide.

Working as a team

As a student or trainee, the rest of the team should be encouraged to feed back about their experiences with you so that, in turn, you can reflect on how you are perceived. Nurses, reception staff and laboratory technicians may be asked to comment on your level of professionalism.

Giving feedback

Occasionally you may be asked to provide feedback on a course or programme. It is important to think objectively about your comments, using the following as a guide:

• Be specific
• Be realistic
• Focus on the issues, not the individuals
• Suggest solutions
• Keep it relevant

23 Medical histories and the presenting complaint

Figure 23.1 Medical history

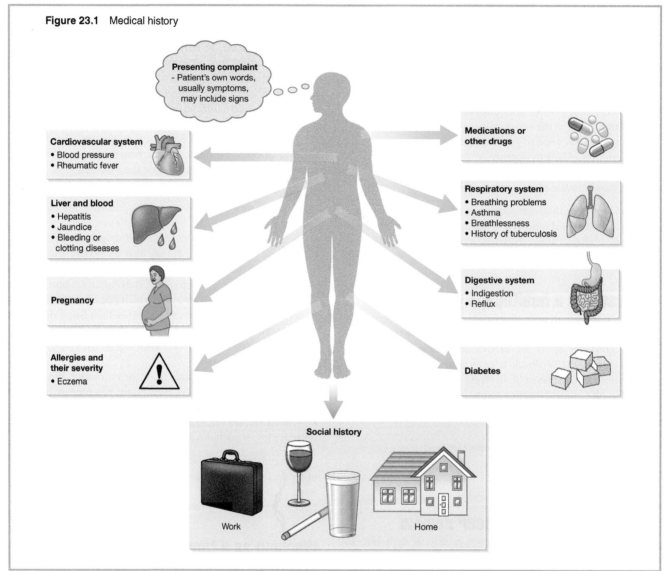

Pre-Clinical Dental Skills at a Glance, First Edition. James Field. © 2016 by John Wiley & Sons, Ltd. Published 2016 by John Wiley & Sons, Ltd.
Companion website: www.wiley.com/go/field/preclinical-dental-skills

An accurate and up-to-date medical history is essential in order to:

• Assess whether your patient is fit enough for you to carry out treatment
• Provide treatment without causing unnecessary complications
• Prescribe medications and anaesthetics appropriately

A medical history is *not* taken solely to determine whether your patient has the potential to transmit an infectious disease; other complications arising from the medical history may also put the patient and the dental team at risk. In addition, a comprehensive medical history may provide an insight into any systemic problems that may manifest themselves in the mouth, such as autoimmune diseases, blood disorders, congenital problems or infections.

On occasion, an accurate medical history may be difficult to take. Patients may be reluctant to divulge their history, especially if the information is sensitive. It is important to remind your patient that the information you record is confidential and to offer them an opportunity to discuss the history further in private. Often patients are given medical history forms to fill in prior to coming into the surgery, which is thought to improve information disclosure. If in doubt, you should always check with your patient's medical practitioner.

Medical history

You should update the record on each occasion that you see your patient. The consultation should be recorded in the notes, including any negative findings. With paper notes there is no need to write out the full medical history on each occasion, although it is a good idea to summarise any significant findings on a regular basis.

Medical problems are most easily divided by bodily system, although it is important to remember that these systems often overlap.

Patients should be encouraged to discuss the following (examples of significant problems are given in brackets):

• Cardiovascular system (myocardial infarction, angina, hypertension, congenital disease or cerebro-vascular events)
• Central nervous system (fits or faints)
• Genitourinary or gastrointestinal (reflux, duodenal/peptic ulcers, Crohn's disease, dysphagia or ulcerative colitis)
• Allergies or sensitivities (drugs or latex)
• Medications
• Respiratory problems (bronchitis, emphysema, asthma, cystic fibrosis, pneumonia, tuberculosis or chronic obstructive pulmonary disease [COPD])
• Endocrine disease (diabetes, thyroid/steroid-based diseases)
• Bleeding abnormalities or blood disorders (haemophilia, anaemia, thalassaemia and leukaemia)
• Infectious diseases (herpes, chickenpox, hepatitis or HIV)
• Musculoskeletal or neurological diseases
• Dermatological disease (eczema, urticaria, psoriasis, lichen planus, pemphigus, pemphigoid, carcinoma/melanoma)
• Liver or kidney disease
• Pregnancy
• Hospital admissions or attendances

As you go through this list, you might want to ask further questions relating to specific medical conditions.

Social history

The social history provides a broad assessment of your patient's well-being. This should at the very least explore the patient's occupation, smoking and alcohol consumption. Occupation may be important due to physiological impacts such as stress, or pathological impacts such as tooth surface loss. It may also be relevant when arranging patient appointments, for example with certain shift patterns or trips away. Smoking has a significant impact on most dental and systemic diseases; an estimate of tobacco intake should be recorded and its form. The GDC makes it the responsibility of everyone involved with your patient's care to emphasise the benefit of smoking cessation. Patients should also be asked to estimate their weekly alcohol intake in units (guidelines for reasonable limits are 14 units per week for women and 21 units per week for men). Any concerns should be raised with the patient and referral should be made to the medical practitioner for possible liver function tests.

It is important, where possible, to enquire about your patient's circumstances at home – is anything significant happening that may be having an impact on their life? If so, it may have consequences for your patient's ability to care for themselves, maintain an upbeat and optimistic approach or deal with bad news.

Previous dental history

The past dental history should enquire about whether your patient is a regular attender and how much dental work they have had carried out before. This can help you to gauge whether any acclimatisation may be required, or how motivated the patient is to maintain their oral health.

Presenting complaint

Where possible, use open questions initially to enquire about your patient's problem. Try to avoid prompting, but then narrow down your questions to address the specific issue. The complaint should be written succinctly, but in the patient's own words; for example, your patient is more likely to complain about a 'broken tooth on the upper right' than a 'fractured 15'.

Pain histories are most common, but your pattern of enquiry could easily relate to other problems such as aesthetics or function:

• Site and location – where does the pain typically present, and does it spread or radiate anywhere?
• What is the nature of the pain – is it sharp or throbbing?
• How long has the problem been present for?
• When did it start or when did you first become aware?
• How long does it last for?
• Does the pain have a gradual onset or is it fairly abrupt?
• Does anything make it better or worse? For example, heat or cold or biting?
• Have you tried painkillers? Are they any help?
• Are there any associated symptoms such as a bad taste, bleeding, swelling or numbness?

At this point you should have sufficient information to proceed with a basic oral health assessment. This will include:

• An extra- and intra-oral examination
• Charting of the hard tissues and the periodontium
• Any special or further investigations
• An assessment of disease risk
• A formal diagnosis
• An initial treatment plan

24 Oral health assessment

Figure 24.1 Oral health assessment

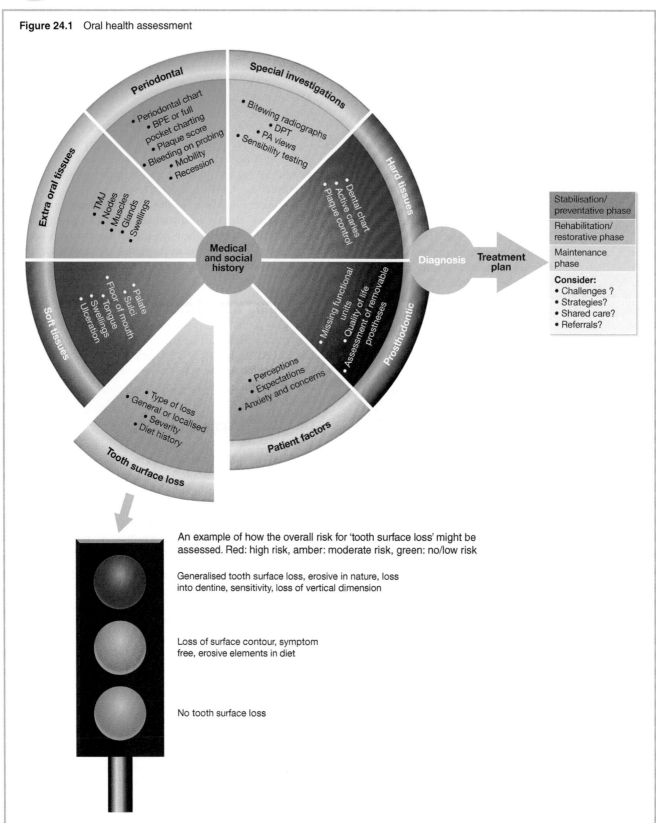

An example of how the overall risk for 'tooth surface loss' might be assessed. Red: high risk, amber: moderate risk, green: no/low risk

Generalised tooth surface loss, erosive in nature, loss into dentine, sensitivity, loss of vertical dimension

Loss of surface contour, symptom free, erosive elements in diet

No tooth surface loss

Pre-Clinical Dental Skills at a Glance, First Edition. James Field. © 2016 by John Wiley & Sons, Ltd. Published 2016 by John Wiley & Sons, Ltd.
Companion website: www.wiley.com/go/field/preclinical-dental-skills

Building on a thorough medical and social history, a comprehensive oral health assessment will allow you to formulate a treatment plan that is specific to your patient's needs. It should emphasise a longer-term preventive approach to care that both the wider dental team and the patient can understand. The assessment should cover several domains, involving examination and history taking, special investigations and a patient-centred dialogue. A level of risk should then be assigned to each of the following:

- Extra-oral
- Intra-oral
  - Soft tissues
  - Hard tissues
  - Periodontal
  - Tooth surface loss
  - Prosthodontic
- Patient-centred factors

Often an oral health assessment template is made available to guide you through this investigative and planning process. Be wary of relying on assessment forms, which are relatively rigid in their format and space allocation; on occasion you may need to make further investigations or record additional information. As always, you must ensure that you record everything you have done, including any negative findings.

Extra-oral assessment

This should include a general assessment of the face, noting any asymmetry, swelling, bruising or paralysis in the facial muscles. It is often easiest to carry out the remainder of this assessment from behind the patient with clean, ungloved hands. Examine the tempero-mandibular joints at the site of the condyles while the patient opens and closes their mouth. Note details of soreness, crepitus, clicking and deviations of the mandible. Palpate the major muscles of mastication for tenderness both within the body and at the insertions; also palpate the submental and submandibular and cervical lymph nodes. Finally, examine the salivary glands for swelling and make a note of whether the presentation is uni- or bilateral.

Soft tissues

A soft tissue assessment should investigate the palate, buccal, labial and lingual sulci and the floor of the mouth. Mirrors should be used to retract the tissues, and if the patient is encouraged to relax the cheeks then vision is greatly improved; a piece of gauze can also be useful wrapped over the tip of the tongue for improved control and better vision of the dorsum, lateral borders and lingual sulci. Intra-oral swellings should be noted along with any signs of ulceration or mucosa of abnormal presentation.

Hard tissues

Chart the teeth and note all carious lesions. Remember that the teeth should be dry and well illuminated to aid in accurate diagnosis. A general assessment of the level of oral hygiene can be made at this stage. The following warrant further investigation:

- Teeth that have been traumatised
- Teeth that are very discoloured
- Teeth that are hypersensitive
- Teeth that are tender to bite on
- Teeth exhibiting fremitus
- Teeth exhibiting fractures or faceting

On occasion it may be appropriate also to record the incisal relationship and the type of occlusal scheme.

Periodontal

The patient's gingival health should be recorded. A Basic Periodontal Examination (BPE) should then be carried out, leading to a full record of periodontal probing depths and bleeding on probing in sextants with signs of pathological pocketing (code ≥3). A plaque score will allow you to provide tailored, effective oral hygiene instruction and serve as a baseline to measure potential progress. Pathological tooth mobility and gingival recession should also be recorded for the entire dentition.

Tooth surface loss

Signs of excessive localised or generalised tooth surface loss should be noted; a range of classifications may be used to record the type, location and severity. It may be necessary to discuss the patient's diet and identify any parafunctional habits.

Prosthodontic

The integrity of both direct and indirect restorative interfaces should be investigated, and recurrent or active caries noted. Record missing functional units along with the presence and type of any removable prostheses. Make an assessment of how partially edentate or completely edentulous patients cope on a day-to-day basis, the quality of their prostheses and the associated edentulous ridges, and the impact of the condition on their quality of life.

Special investigations

At this stage, you may want to make further investigations to help you arrive at a definitive diagnosis. These may include vitality testing, radiographs (to assess bone levels, caries, periodontal pathology and resorption) or a diet history.

Staged treatment plan

Once the information has been collated, it is important to identify any particular challenges to providing treatment. This may relate to the patient themselves (for example in terms of motivation, attendance pattern or medical history) or the specific treatment (for example most teeth being of poor prognosis, or no previous denture-wearing experience). Appropriate treatment strategies should be identified, and shared care or referral considered where appropriate. The treatment plan should be clearly split into three stages:

- Stabilisation and prevention
- Restoration and rehabilitation
- Review and maintenance

Patient-centred factors and diagnoses

You should have kept the patient informed and included along your investigative journey, and you should now allocate suitable time to discussing your definitive diagnoses and treatment options. Record that the options and alternatives have been discussed, and make sure that the patient understands the advantages and risks of each approach. Obtain written or verbal consent for treatment and record the details accurately in the notes before you begin.

25 Charting the dentition

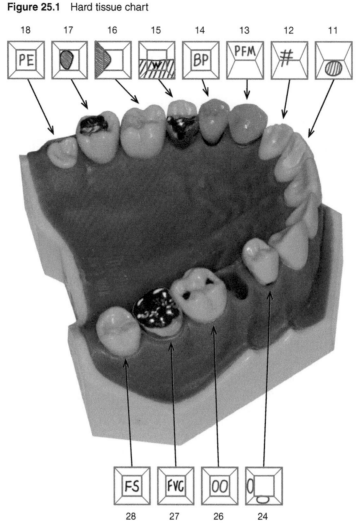

Figure 25.1   Hard tissue chart

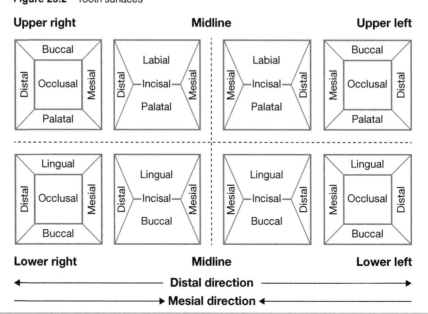

Figure 25.2   Tooth surfaces

Pre-Clinical Dental Skills at a Glance, First Edition. James Field. © 2016 by John Wiley & Sons, Ltd. Published 2016 by John Wiley & Sons, Ltd.
Companion website: www.wiley.com/go/field/preclinical-dental-skills

Being able to compile a dental chart is critical for accurate record keeping and treatment planning. The chart forms part of the health record and so it is recognised as a legal document. It represents a patient's full dentition, illustrating each tooth surface and whether it is restored or in need of restoration. When updated at each review, the chart provides a record of past treatment as well as an accurate contemporaneous record.

It is important to be able to identify individual teeth and visualise them in a dry, well-lit field. It is also useful to have a standardised approach, understood by those who will be noting down your findings; often this will be your nurse, but while at dental school it may be a colleague or a supervisor. Although someone else may be compiling the chart, its accuracy is still your responsibility. On the first few occasions that you work with a particular individual, it is a good idea to stop periodically to check the record – or even to cast your eye over the whole chart once you have finished.

Completion of the chart may be delayed until further investigations such as radiographs have been taken and reported.

Tooth notations

Tooth notations are used to identify individual teeth. The Federation Dentaire Internationale (FDI) notation is used most commonly in Europe. This two-digit system starts with the first incisor in the patient's upper right quadrant and progresses distally before moving on to the next quadrant in a clockwise motion. The first number identifies the quadrant, while the second number identifies the individual tooth.

You may occasionally come across the older Zigmondy–Palmer notation, which uses a pictorial grid, negating the need for the first digit in the equivalent FDI notation. For example, |3 would become 23 in the FDI notation. FDI superseded this notation because it was easier to pronounce in conversation and dictation and more readily communicable in print.

Pictorial charts

Although each tooth could be detailed in written form within the clinical notes, the pictorial chart offers expedience while recording and reviewing the record. Each tooth should be charted with a recognised symbol that denotes the status of the tooth. A pictorial chart is normally laid out as a flat rectangular chart representing the teeth as viewed from the front of the patient; the left-hand side of the chart represents the patient's right-hand side. Each tooth comprises five surfaces; posterior teeth differ to incisors and canines in that they present with an occlusal surface rather than an incisal edge.

- Mesial indicates a proximity to the front (anterior) of the mouth.
- Distal indicates a proximity to the back (posterior) of the mouth.
- Labial indicates a proximity to the lip.
- Buccal indicates a proximity to the cheek.
- Palatal indicates a proximity to the palate.
- Lingual indicates a proximity to the tongue.

Most of the common notations are shown in Figure 25.2.

Periodontal examination

Recording details of the supporting structures of the teeth is important for diagnosing, managing and monitoring periodontal conditions; however, this information is also vitally impotant when planning treatment, particularly the restorative phase. The patient's plaque control and plaque score can also be recorded, the latter proving useful for tailored oral hygiene advice and as a motivational tool. Pathological mobility and gingival recession should be recorded when present.

The basic periodontal examination is a useful screening tool and employs a dedicated probe (the World Health Organisation probe). This probe has a ball-shaped tip and a black band of between 3.5 mm and 5.5 mm; these features allow grading of subgingival calculus/overhangs and pathological pocketing, respectively. The mouth is divided into sextants, and the probe should be walked gently around the gingival sulci within each sextant, noting down the highest score recorded from the BPE criteria.

A BPE score of 3 or more within a particular sextant indicates the need for a full individual pocket chart within that sextant. Whether the periodontal pockets bleed on probing (BOP) should also be recorded.

BPE scoring codes:

0 Black band completely visible, no BOP, no calculus/overhangs
1 Black band completely visible but BOP, no calculus/overhangs
2 Black band completely visible, but calculus/overhangs
3 Black band partially visible
4 Black band entirely within pocket
* Furcation involvement

26 Delivering oral hygiene instructions

Figure 26.1 Oral hygiene instructions

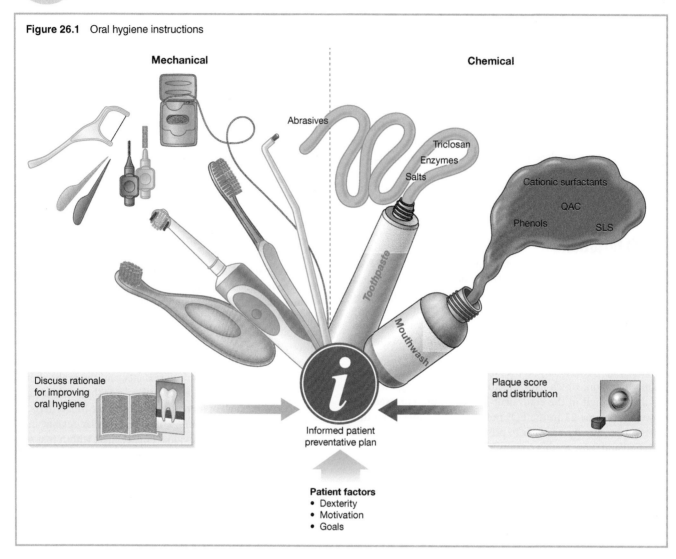

The delivery of oral hygiene instructions should form part of an overall patient-centred preventive plan. This will necessarily include:

- Empowering the patient, by ensuring that they understand how plaque control works and why it is necessary
- Ensuring that the patient knows about suitable methods of mechanical and chemical plaque control
- Gauging the patient's level of dexterity and motivation and identifying any relevant personal goals
- Initiating, mediating or delivering smoking cessation support, where relevant
- Professional scaling and prophylaxis to a level that the patient would otherwise find difficult or impossible to achieve

Assess needs and examine practice

In order to devise a tailored preventive plan, it is necessary to enquire about your patient's existing oral hygiene practices; part of this is about determining whether they are actually effective (regardless of the number of times each day that your patient cleans their teeth). This will involve disclosing the patient's existing plaque so that you can identify both the amount and location(s) of plaque deposits. It is also worthwhile asking your patient then to clean their teeth, so that together you can identify areas that are being missed. It is essential to involve your patient, demonstrating and explaining your findings as you proceed. Your patient needs to understand the basic mechanisms of oral disease and the effects of an undisturbed biofilm. The challenge for you as a healthcare professional is to convey this information in a simple and accessible way. Comprehensive notes should be made so that you can track your patient's progress.

Plan

Once you have an idea of what is required, you can draw up a tailored preventive plan. You should consider how motivated your patient is; it may be helpful at this stage to reiterate any personal goals that your patient may have and how compliance will increase the chances of reaching them. Other considerations are your patient's dexterity and level of competence. On occasion your patient may be cared for by another person, so that person too should be at the centre of your discussion.

Implement and review

Once you are happy that an effective plan has been devised and accepted, it is important to move forward in a timely manner. Give the patient an opportunity to implement the necessary changes to their oral hygiene regime, but review the situation again relatively soon to ensure that they are adopting the new measures effectively. It is sometimes a good idea to provide the patient with some disclosing tablets for use at home so that they can monitor their own oral hygiene efforts between appointments. Concurrently other preventive regimes should be put into place, such as support for smoking cessation and supportive therapies such as scaling and root debridement.

Mechanical control of plaque

Ideally, the teeth should be brushed once in the morning and once in the evening, for approximately two minutes on each occasion. If your patient consumes relatively acidic foods and drinks for breakfast, then it may be beneficial for them to brush beforehand and simply use a fluoride mouthwash afterwards.

A wide range of brushes are available. A good manual brush should have medium to soft bristles. There is no real need to have a hard-bristled brush; they may traumatise the soft tissues and are less likely to adapt to the hard and soft tissue contour. Similarly, the brush head size should not be too large – around the size of your little finger from knuckle to tip is about right. When the bristles start to splay, it is time to replace the brush. Children and babies should have their teeth brushed as soon as they are able, using appropriate toothpaste. Infant brushes are usually smaller in size with a novelty or chunky handle to facilitate the early stages of holding the brush by themselves.

A number of brushing techniques exist, the majority of which are based around a short back-and-forth motion with the brush head at a particular angle to the tooth surfaces (usually at 45 degrees with bristles pointing in an apical direction; the 'Bass' technique). Modifications to the technique include a 'roll' or 'flick' up and away from the gingival margin, which is thought to help debride the area. It is important to demonstrate this action on a model so that your patient understands the mechanics of how the technique works. Powered brushes are available with a circular reciprocating head, or an ultrasonic head. There is mixed evidence about whether they are more effective than manual brushes – however, there is definitely a novelty value, especially with children, and this may go a long way to improving motivation. These types of brushes can be invaluable for people with limited dexterity or poor access to the oral cavity. Although toothpastes often have a significant level of chemical activity, they also provide an essential lubricative and foaming action, which helps the brush to contact the tissues and debride the area.

The interproximal areas of teeth represent a significant portion of the total coronal surface area; they are also most likely to retain food debris and develop as areas of stagnation. Interdental cleaning is therefore extremely important and, although it does not need to be carried out every day, it should be done effectively. A range of products exist including floss, brushes, wedges/sticks and water jets. Most of the time the most relevant aid depends on patient preference, dexterity and anatomy. Floss is sold as waxed or unwaxed, threaded or as a tape; for tight contacts the waxed tape is often easier to use. The floss should be wrapped around the third finger of each hand, leaving the thumb and forefinger free to introduce the floss through the contact area. Importantly, once in the embrasure space, floss should be pulled mesially and distally against each proximal surface rather than simply 'jiggled' up and down, which can traumatise the interdental tissues. Variants are available with rigid elements for passing under appliances or pontics, and a thicker area for actively cleaning under pontics. Bottle brushes are useful when the embrasure space is too large for floss to be effective, but too small for a conventional brush. They are also extremely useful in class 3 furcation lesions.

Chemical control of plaque

Some toothpastes contain chemically active compounds such as enzyme systems, antimicrobials or heavy metal salts. However, it is the mouthwashes that contain the largest range of chemicals for controlling plaque. Some are targeted at preventing the proliferation of a biofilm such as cationic surfactants (chlorhexidine), quaternary ammonium compounds (cetyl pyridinium chloride in Aquafresh and Dentyl pH), phenols (thymol in Listerine) and Triclosan (Colgate Total and Plax). Others are targeted at preventing the aggregation and adherence of plaque, such as sodium lauryl sulphate (Plax). It is worth considering the full range of these chemicals when devising a tailored oral health regime, to be used at times other than brushing. Chlorhexidine should only be used in the shorter term until effective plaque control has been established; there are issues with staining and taste disturbance if it is used for longer.

27 Offering smoking cessation advice

Figure 27.1 Smoking cessation advice

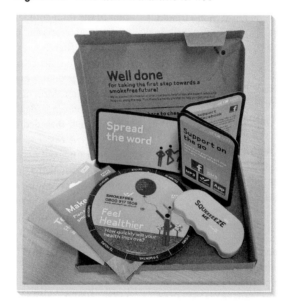

Figure 27.2 NHS Quit Kit available for free

At the time of writing, according to ASH (Action on Smoking and Health), there are around 10 million smokers in Great Britain and a further 15 million ex-smokers. Aside from the wider health implications, smoking is a major risk factor for periodontal disease and oral cancers. ASH estimates that around 70% of current smokers would like to give up smoking altogether, which means that there are around 7 million people who would undoubtedly benefit in some way from smoking cessation advice.

Why should dentists offer this advice?

As dentists we are unusual in that we recall patients for assessment on a regular basis. This provides an excellent opportunity not only to monitor for oral disease, but repeatedly to offer an intervention such as support for smoking cessation. Furthermore, as a dental team we already possess many of the skills required in order to communicate information effectively and modify patient behaviour.

Stages of smoking cessation

The smoking cessation model shown in Figure 27.1 identifies a smoker as 'content' or 'concerned'. Often the contented smoker is unaware of the significant health risks associated with smoking, or is unwilling to accept that those issues relate to them at that moment in time. As a smoker starts to internalise the health risks and accepts that smoking is damaging their health, they will become 'concerned'; although they are still smoking at this stage, this type of patient will usually be very receptive to a smoking cessation intervention that results in a quit plan and/or counselling. Hopefully the intervention will result in behaviours that reduce or eliminate the smoking habit. Once this has been achieved, it is important for the patient to remain a non-smoker – and this stage is therefore often considered to be critical.

As busy healthcare professionals it can be hard to find time to squeeze in an intervention such as smoking cessation. However, a simple 30-second model exists providing a framework through which we can make enquiries and provide advice about smoking cessation in a logical and structured way. This model is often known as the '3 As'.

Ask

At the very least, we should be routinely recording whether or not our patients smoke as part of a comprehensive medical and social history.

You may wish to make further enquiries about your patient's smoking habit:

- Exactly how much does your patient smoke and in what form?
- For how long has your patient smoked?
- Has your patient ever stopped smoking?
- How does your patient feel about stopping smoking?

Advise

It can be impossible at this stage to judge whether your patient may be a 'content' or a 'concerned' smoker. As such, it is appropriate to spend a moment highlighting the benefits of quitting. In relation to oral health these may include:

- Reducing the likelihood of periodontal disease and oral cancers
- Improved outcomes of periodontal treatment
- Improved taste and smell
- Better saliva flow and quality

Try to get your patient to identify their own reasons for quitting. Help them to recognise the wider health benefits of quitting:

- Breathing is easier
- Circulation improves
- Risk of heart attack and lung cancer reduces
- Financial benefits

Even brief advice can result in the concerned smoker becoming motivated enough to quit. Contented smokers are harder to convince, so it is important to make your advice clear, unambiguous and personalised. If your patient believes that your advice has personal relevance, then it will have a greater motivational impact. Sometimes it is also useful to try to investigate any perceived barriers to quitting. Do not merely offer advice on one occasion; it may take several attempts before your patient becomes convinced or motivated enough to quit. As always, record your discussions and outcomes in the notes.

Interactive online resources can be extremely useful for patients to access in their own time, such as http://smokefree.nhs.uk. There patients can find:

- Ways to quit
- Real-life successful case stories
- Advice and information
- Access to national and local helplines
- Online chats with an expert
- Addiction tests and cost calculators
- Free 'quit kits' and Quit apps for mobile devices
- Support communities and discussion fora
- Support for 'at risk' groups such as pregnant women

Act

Once your patient feels motivated enough to try smoking cessation, you should refer them to an intensive support service such as NHS Stop Smoking Services. Patients often ask what will happen next, so you should know what tools are available:

Non-pharmacological
- Willpower and self-help material
- Cognitive behaviour therapy
- Hypnotics
- Acupuncture

Pharmacological
- Nicotine replacement therapy:
  - Patches
  - Inhalers
  - Gum
  - Lozenges
  - Nasal sprays
  - Microtabs (under tongue)
- Bupropion (Zyban®) – prescription only
- Varenicline (Champix®) – prescription only

28 Requesting and reporting on intra-oral radiographs

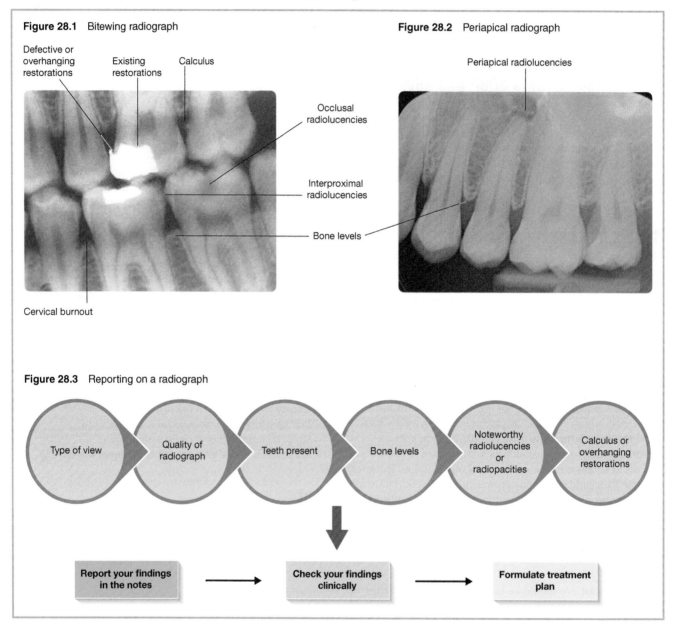

Figure 28.1 Bitewing radiograph

- Defective or overhanging restorations
- Existing restorations
- Calculus
- Occlusal radiolucencies
- Interproximal radiolucencies
- Bone levels
- Cervical burnout

Figure 28.2 Periapical radiograph

- Periapical radiolucencies

Figure 28.3 Reporting on a radiograph

Type of view → Quality of radiograph → Teeth present → Bone levels → Noteworthy radiolucencies or radiopacities → Calculus or overhanging restorations

Report your findings in the notes → Check your findings clinically → Formulate treatment plan

Pre-Clinical Dental Skills at a Glance, First Edition. James Field. © 2016 by John Wiley & Sons, Ltd. Published 2016 by John Wiley & Sons, Ltd.
Companion website: www.wiley.com/go/field/preclinical-dental-skills

adiographs provide invaluable supplementary information when investigating hard and soft tissue pathology, bone levels, tooth/root position or anatomy, and trauma. They are also used routinely for endodontic treatments. A comprehensive list of indications and intervals for taking radiographs is provided by the Faculty of General Dental Practitioners in their guide 'Selection Criteria for Dental Radiography'.

In all likelihood as a practitioner in primary care, you will be taking radiographs yourself. It is therefore important to know *how* to take a radiograph, the details of which are not within the scope of this chapter, which offers background information.

While working in a secondary care setting with a separate radiology department, or if making a referral for a radiograph elsewhere, you will need to make an appropriate request for the radiographs to be taken. Two important pieces of legislation ensure that quality assurance processes are followed and dosages are kept as low as practicable.

Ionising Radiation Regulations 1999

Often referred to as IRR, these regulations exist to protect the dental team and the public. In the main they refer to the maintenance and safe operation of radiography equipment, and controlling the areas in which that equipment operates. The IRR support the implementation of local rules that quality assure radiographic processes and provide adequate assessment of any potential risks.

Ionising Radiation (Medical Exposure) Regulations 2000

Often referred to as IRMER, this more recent legislation is concerned primarily with patient safety. It is about ensuring that doses are effective but as low as practicable. The patient's exposure should be considered in light of the diagnostic benefit – so in other words, you should be able to justify your decision to take the radiograph. Once you have decided to go ahead, the legislation also ensures that you are taking effective steps to reduce the dose; for example, using rectangular collimation and a fast film. IRMER also designates certain roles to the team; for example, the practitioner making the referral for the radiograph and the operator taking the radiograph. Often in primary care these roles are carried out by the same person. Nonetheless, practitioners and operators must have sufficient training in radiology and radiography.

Making a request

If someone other than you will be taking the radiograph, then a suitable request should be recorded. This request should include:

- Patient details
- Justification for taking the radiograph(s)
- Date of the last radiograph
- Details of the referrer
- Which views are to be taken

The operator should then also record their details, which views were taken and the number of attempts.

Reporting

There is an obligation to record the radiographic findings in the written notes, as well as storing the radiographic image securely. Measures should be put into place that allow errors or faults to be recorded and acted on, and radiographs and their reports to be audited.

A radiograph report should address the following:

- View(s) taken
- Quality of the radiograph (see Further reading)
- Teeth present, both erupted and unerupted
- Bone levels/bony support for the teeth
- Presence and location of calculus
- Noteworthy radiolucencies and radiopacities
- Existing restorations

Tips for reporting

It is helpful to have a consistent approach to reporting. The report needs to be comprehensive enough that if the radiographic image were lost, there would be no significant detriment to the patient's care.

The first task is to ensure that you are reporting on the correct image; check the patient's details. Try not to dive straight in to the area of concern – be comprehensive and structured. It is very easy to miss other problems if you do not maintain a standardised approach.

Reporting on radiographs is relatively easy – say what you see! At times, however, the task can seem harder, because the assumption often is that a diagnosis can be made from the radiographic image alone. It is important to remember that you cannot report caries or pathology from a 2D radiographic image –you can only report on radiolucent or radiopaque features that are then checked clinically before a diagnosis is confirmed. Be mindful that tooth morphology and tooth position can both result in radiographic features that may be mistaken for caries. Familiarise yourself with the concept of burnout, as this will often lead you to think that there are pathological processes happening at the boundaries between relatively radiopaque and radiolucent structures.

Try to refrain from calling radiographs 'x-rays'; while x-rays are used to create the diagnostic image, they are invisible to the naked eye.

Further reading

Chapter 1
Bonehill, JA (2010) *Managing Health and Safety in the Dental Practice: A Practical Guide*, Chichester: John Wiley & Sons.

GDC (2013) *Standards for the Dental Team*, London: General Dental Council, available at http://www.gdc-uk.org/

GDC (2013) *Scope of Practice*, London: General Dental Council, available at http://www.gdc-uk.org/

Rattan, R, Chambers, R & Wakley, G (2002) *Clinical Governance in General Dental Practice*, Milton Keynes: Radcliffe Publishing.

Chapter 2
Field, J & Vernazza, C (2013) Developing a grading matrix for reflection, *Medical Education* 47(5): 531.

GDC (2013) *Continuing Professional Development for Dental Professionals*, London: General Dental Council, available at http://www.gdc-uk.org/

London, M (ed.) (2011) *The Oxford Handbook of Lifelong Learning*, New York: Oxford University Press.

Moon, JA (2006) *Learning Journals: A Handbook for Reflective Practice and Professional Development*, London: Routledge.

Chapter 3
Berkovitz, BKB, Holland, GR & Moxham, BJ (2009) *Oral Anatomy, Histology and Embryology*, 4th edn, St Louis, MO: Mosby, Chapter on 'Dento-osseous structures'.

Chapter 4
Banerjee, A & Watson, TF (2011) *Pickard's Manual of Operative Dentistry*, 9th edn, Oxford: Oxford University Press, Chapter 5.8.

Scheller-Sheridan, C (2011) *Basic Guide to Dental Instruments*, Oxford: Wiley-Blackwell.

Summit, JB, Robbins, JW, Hilton, TJ & Schwartz, RS (eds) (2006) *Fundamentals of Operative Dentistry: A Contemporary Approach*, Hanover Park, IL: Quintessence, Chapter 6.

Chapter 5
Banerjee, A & Watson, TF (2011) *Pickard's Manual of Operative Dentistry*, 9th edn, Oxford: Oxford University Press, Chapter 5.8.2.

Mount, GJ & Hume, WR (1998) *Preservation and Restoration of Tooth Structure*, St Louis, MO: Mosby, Chapter 6.

Chapter 6
Gandavadi, A, Ramsay, JRE & Burke, FJT (2007) Assessment of dental student posture in two seating positions using RULA methodology – a pilot study, *British Dental Journal* 203(10): 601–605.

Chapter 7
Summit, JB, Robbins, JW, Hilton, TJ & Schwartz, RS (eds) (2006) *Fundamentals of Operative Dentistry: A Contemporary Approach*, Hanover Park, IL: Quintessence, p. 366.

Chapter 9
Andlaw, RJ & Rock, WP (1998) *A Manual of Paediatric Dentistry*, 4th edn, St Louis, MO: Churchill Livingstone, Chapter 8.

Arana-Chavez, VE & Massa, LF (2004) Odontoblasts: The cells forming and maintaining dentine, *International Journal of Biochemistry and Cell Biology* 36(8): 1367–1373.

Banerjee, A (2013) Minimal intervention dentistry: Part 7. Minimally invasive operative caries management: Rationale and techniques, *British Dental Journal* 214: 107–111.

Ricketts, DN, Kidd, EA, Innes, N & Clarkson, J (2006) Towards the pulp – complete or ultraconservative removal of decayed tissue in unfilled teeth, *Cochrane Database of Systematic Reviews* 19(3), CD003808.

Chapter 10
Banerjee, A & Watson, TF (2011) *Pickard's Manual of Operative Dentistry*, 9th edn, Oxford: Oxford University Press, Chapter 5.10.

Chapter 11
Banerjee, A & Watson, TF (2011) *Pickard's Manual of Operative Dentistry*, 9th edn, Oxford: Oxford University Press, Chapter 7.7.

Chapter 12
Whitworth, JM (2002) *Rational Root Canal Treatment in Practice*, Hanover Park, IL: Quintessence, Chapter 4.

Chapter 13
Summit, JB, Robbins, JW, Hilton, TJ & Schwartz, RS (eds) (2006) *Fundamentals of Operative Dentistry: A Contemporary Approach*, Hanover Park, IL: Quintessence, pp. 377–379.

Chapter 15
Mount, GJ & Hume, WR (1998) *Preservation and Restoration of Tooth Structure*, St Louis, MO: Mosby, Chapter 8.

Chapter 16
Burkard, H (2009) *Esthetics with Resin Composite: Basics and Techniques*, Hanover Park, IL: Quintessence.

Chapter 17
Heasman, P, Preshaw, P, Robertson, P & Chapple, I (2004) *Successful Periodontal Therapy: A Non-surgical Approach*, Hanover Park, IL: Quintessence, Chapter 3.

Chapter 18
Banerjee, A & Watson, TF (2011) *Pickard's Manual of Operative Dentistry*, 9th edn, Oxford: Oxford University Press, Chapter 5.6.

Carrotte, P (2004) Endodontics: Part 6. Rubber dam and access cavities, *British Dental Journal* 197: 527–534.

Chapter 19

Correll, R (2013) *Digital SLR Photography All-in-One For Dummies*, Chichester: John Wiley & Sons.

Wassell, R, Naru, A, Steele, J & Nohl, F (2008) *Applied Occlusion*, Hanover Park, IL: Quintessence, Chapters 8.1–8.6.

Wassell, R, Walls, AWG, Steele, J & Nohl, F (2002) *A Clinical Guide to Crowns and Other Extra-coronal Restorations*, London: British Dental Journal, pp. 46–51.

Chapter 20

Pankhurst, C & Coulter, W (2009) *Basic Guide to Infection Prevention and Control in Dentistry*, Oxford: Wiley-Blackwell.

Chapter 21

Hadden, A, Eaton, K, Ormond, C, Holt, V & Ladwa, R (eds) (2009) *Clinical Examination and Record Keeping*, London: Faculty of General Dental Practitioners.

Harrison, C, Hart, J & Wass, V (2007) Learning to communicate using the Calgary–Cambridge framework, *The Clinical Teacher* 4(3): 159–164.

Lillyman, S & Merrix, P (2012) *Nursing and Health Record Keeping: Survival Guide*, London: Routledge.

Chapter 22

Delany, C & Molloy, E (eds) (2009) *Clinical Education in the Health Professions: An Educator's Guide*, St Louis, MO: Churchill Livingstone, Chapter 8.

Chapter 23

Greenwood, M & Corbett, I (eds) (2012) *Dental Emergencies*, Oxford: Wiley-Blackwell, Chapters 3, 11–12.

Porter, ST, Scully, C, Welsby, PD & Gleeson, M (1999) *Medicine and Surgery for Dentistry*, 2nd edn, St Louis, MO: Churchill Livingstone.

Scully, C (2010) *Medical Problems in Dentistry*, 6th edn, St Louis, MO: Churchill Livingstone, Chapter 1.

Chapter 24

Andlaw, RJ & Rock, WP (1998) *A Manual of Paediatric Dentistry*, 4th edn, St Louis, MO: Churchill Livingstone, Chapter 1.4.

Basker, RM, Davenport, JC & Thomason, JM (2011) *Prosthetic Treatment of the Edentulous Patient*, 5th edn, Oxford: Wiley-Blackwell, Chapter 7.

Horner, K & Eaton, K (eds) (2013) *Selection Criteria for Dental Radiography*, London: Faculty of General Dental Practice.

Laney, WR, Salinas, TJ, Carr, AB, Sreenivas, K & Eckert, SE (eds) (2011) *Diagnosis and Treatment in Prosthodontics*, 2nd edn, Hanover Park, IL: Quintessence, pp. 22–37.

Moore, UJ (2011) *Principles of Oral and Maxillofacial Surgery*, 6th edn, Oxford: Wiley-Blackwell, Chapter 1.

Palmer RM & Floyd, PD (2003) *A Clinical Guide to Periodontology*, 2nd edn, London: British Dental Journal, Chapter 1.

Zarb, GA, Hobkirk, J, Eckert, S & Jacob, R (2012) *Prosthodontic Treatment for Edentulous Patients*, 13th edn, St Louis, MO: Mosby, Chapter 5.

Chapter 25

Hollins, C (2013) *Levison's Textbook for Dental Nurses*, Oxford: Wiley-Blackwell, Chapter 12.

Miller, M & Scully, C (2011) *Mosby's Textbook of Dental Nursing*, St Louis, MO: Mosby, Chapter 7.

Chapter 26

Heasman, P, Preshaw, P, Robertson, P & Chapple, I (2004) *Successful Periodontal Therapy: A Non-surgical Approach*, Hanover Park, IL: Quintessence, Chapter 2.

Chapter 27

ASH, Action on Smoking and Health, www.ash.org.uk

Carr, A & Ebbert, J (2012) Interventions for tobacco cessation in the dental setting, *Cochrane Database of Systematic Reviews*, 6.

Smokefree, www.nhs.uk/smokefree

Chapter 28

Horner, K & Eaton, KA (eds) (2013) *Selection Criteria for Dental Radiography*, 3rd edn, London: Faculty of General Dental Practice.

Horner, K, Rout, J & Rushton, VE (2003) *Interpreting Dental Radiographs*, Hanover Park, IL: Quintessence.

Whaites, E (2002) *Essentials of Dental Radiography and Radiology*, 3rd edn, St Louis, MO: Churchill Livingstone, Chapter 6.

Index

Pre-Clinical Dental Skills at a Glance, First Edition. James Field. © 2016 by John Wiley & Sons, Ltd. Published 2016 by John Wiley & Sons, Ltd.
Companion website: www.wiley.com/go/field/preclinical-dental-skills